# Abstracts of the Third International Symposium on Inborn Errors of Metabolism in Humans

Munich, March 7–9, 1984

KARGER

S. Karger · Basel · München · Paris · London · New York · Tokyo · Sydney

Printed in Germany
ISBN 3–8055–3894–4

## Local Organizing Committee

| | |
|---|---|
| Chairman | Professor Dr. N. Zöllner |
| Secretary | Professor Dr. G. Wolfram |
| Members | Priv.-Doz. Dr. O. Adam |
| | Priv.-Doz. Dr. H. Dörfler |
| | Priv.-Doz. Dr. Ch. Keller |
| | Priv.-Doz. Dr. F. Spengel |
| | Dr. U. Sprandel |

## Local Scientific Committee

Professor Dr. H. Cleve
Professor Dr. W. Forth
Professor Dr. W. Gutensohn
Professor Dr. G. Riethmüller
Professor Dr. G. Wolfram
Professor Dr. H. G. Zachau
Professor Dr. N. Zöllner

## International Scientific Committee

| | |
|---|---|
| H. Aebi † | Switzerland |
| H. Bickel | W. Germany |
| H. Cleve | W. Germany |
| F. Cockburn | Great Britain |
| L. J. Elsas | U.S.A. |
| W. Forth | W. Germany |
| J. Frézal | France |
| R. Gitzelmann | Switzerland |
| W. Gröbner | W. Germany |
| W. Gutensohn | W. Germany |
| J. B. Holton | Great Britain |
| F. van Hoof | Belgium |
| J. T. Ireland | Great Britain |
| N. Kretchmer | U.S.A. |
| W. L. Nyhan | U.S.A. |
| G. Riethmüller | W. Germany |
| J. E. Seegmüller | U.S.A. |
| O. Sperling | Israel |
| H. F. Woods | Great Britain |
| R. W. E. Watts | Great Britain |
| G. Wolfram | W. Germany |
| H. G. Zachau | W. Germany |
| N. Zöllner | W. Germany |

## Acknowledgements

The local organizers gratefully acknowledge the generous support of the Deutsche Forschungsgemeinschaft, the Bayerische Staatsministerium für Unterricht und Kultus and the Landeshauptstadt München.

The Symposium is held under the patronage of the Bavarian Government and the auspices of the University of Munich.

In addition, our thanks are due to the Following for valued contributions (situation at printing time):

Wellcome, Großburgwedel
Travenol, München
Holphar, St. Ingbert
Merck, Darmstadt
Bayer, Leverkusen
Milupa, Friedrichsdorf
Madaus, Köln
Boehringer, Mannheim
Nourypharma, München
Sandoz, Nürnberg
Farmitalia, Freiburg
Karger, Basel
Knoll, Ludwigshafen
Lilly, Bad Homburg
Paul-Martini-Stiftung, Mainz
Röhm, Weiterstadt
Hoechst, Frankfurt
Nattermann, Köln
Immuno, Heidelberg

## General Information

### Location

The symposium will be held in the lecture hall and rooms of the Pharmacological Institute of the University of Munich, Nußbaumstraße 26, 8000 München 2 (FRG). 10 minutes walking distance from Central Station; 8 minutes walking from center ot the town; 3 minutes to underground-station.

### Public Transportation

Munich has a well organized public transportation system with U-Bahn, S-Bahn, busses, and taxi. If you come by plane either take a taxi (approx. price DM 30.-) or take the airport bus (price DM 5.-) to the Central Station.

### Congress Office

During the symposium:

Pharmacological Institute
Nußbaumstraße 26, from 8 a.m. - 6 p.m.
Telephone: (089) 5384-244
(dial through)

Before the symposium:

Medical Polyclinic
Pettenkoferstraße 8a
Telephone:
(089) 5160-3500

### Presentations

Official language of the symposium will be English, free communications also in German or French, but slides must be in English. For free communications 10 min speaking time and 5 min discussion. Equipment for the projection of 5x5 cm (36 mm) slides will be available.

## Social Programme

### Tuesday, March 6, 1984

| | |
|---|---|
| Noon–20.00 | Registration at the lecture hall Pharmacological Institute. After 18.00 coffee or beer and snacks will be offered at an informal get together. |

### Wednesday, March 7, 1984

| | |
|---|---|
| 14.30 | City tour with visit to Nymphenburg castle. For starting point please contact congress office. |
| 19.00 | Traditional Ash-Wednesday fish-dinner, "Ratskeller", Marienplatz |

### Thursday, March 8, 1984

| | |
|---|---|
| 14.00 | Walk through old Munich with a guide. For starting point please contact congress office. |
| 19.00 | Reception by the Government of Bavaria<br>Residenz, Residenzplatz.<br>For details please contact congress office |

### Friday, March 9, 1984

| | |
|---|---|
| 9.00 | Alte and Neue Pinakothek (state galleries). For details please contact congress office |

# Scientific Programme

## Wednesday, March 7, 1984

| | 9.00 – 12.30 | | 14.00 – 17.00 |
|---|---|---|---|
| Room A | *Main Session 1*<br>Inborn Errors of the Adult | | *Main Session 2*<br>Molecular Mechanisms |
| Room B | *Short Communications*<br>Molecular Mechanisms | | *Short Communications*<br>Inborn Errors of the Adult |
| Room C | | | *Short Communications*<br>Genetic Counselling |

## Thursday, March 8, 1984

| | | | |
|---|---|---|---|
| Room A | *Main Session 3*<br>Genetic Counselling | | *Main Session 4*<br>Pharmacogenetics |
| Room B | *Short Communications*<br>Pharmacogenetics | | *Short Communications*<br>Inborn Errors of the Adult |
| Room C | *Short Communications*<br>Molecular Mechanisms | | *Short Communications*<br>Nutrition and Genetic Disease<br>Late Comers' Session I |

## Friday, March 9, 1984

| | | | |
|---|---|---|---|
| Room A | *Main Session 5*<br>Immunogenetics | | *Main Session 6*<br>Nutrition and Genetics Disease |
| Room B | *Short Communications*<br>Nutrition and Genetic Disease | | |
| Room C | *Short Communications*<br>Late Comers' Session II | | |

## **Scientific Programme,** Room A

WEDNESDAY, MARCH 7, 1984

| | |
|---|---|
| 8.45 - 9.00 | Opening without Ceremony |
| 9.00 -12.30 | Session 1 |

INBORN ERRORS OF THE ADULT

Chairmen: R.W.E. Watts (Harrow/UK)
N. Zöllner (München/FRG)

U. Beisiegel (Marburg/FRG)
Familial Hypercholesterolemia - Multiple Mutations at the LDL-Receptor Locus

K. Sandhoff (Bonn/FRG)
Gangliosidoses: Function and Relevance of Activator Proteins

10.30-11.00 Coffee Break

K. von Figura (Münster/FRG)
Pathogenesis of Late Manifestation of Metachromatic Leucodystrophy

M.F. Niermeijer (Rotterdam/Holland)
Glykogenosis Type II, the Origin of Early and Late Forms

Lunch

---

14.00-17.30 Session 2

MOLECULAR MECHANISMS

Chairmen: K. Betke (München/FRG)
H.G. Zachau (München/FRG)

W. Hörz (München /FRG)
Human Genes at the Molecular Level

A.W. Nienhuis (Bethesda/USA)
The Thalassemias: Molecular Mechanism and Treatment by Fetal Gene Activation

15.30-16.00 Coffee Break

R. Williamson (London/UK)
The Use of Random Cloned Genes to Find the Defect in Muscular Dystrophy

M.F. Perutz, D.J. Abraham (Cambridge/UK)
A Crystallographic Approach to the Development of Drugs against Sickle Cell Anaemia

## Room A

THURSDAY, MARCH 8, 1984

| | |
|---|---|
| 9.00–12.00 | Session 3 |
| | **GENETIC COUNSELLING – TRENDS AND PERSPECTIVES** |
| | Chairmen: O. Sperling (Tel Aviv/Israel) |
| | H. Cleve (München/FRG) |
| | F. Vogel (Heidelberg/FRG) |
| | General Problems of Genetic Counselling |
| | G. Utermann (Marburg/FRG) |
| | Lipoprotein Analysis and Counselling in Arteriosclerotic Diseases |
| 10.30–11.00 | Coffee Break |
| | H.H. Ropers (Freiburg/FRG) |
| | DNA-Analysis in Genetic Counselling |
| | Lunch |
| 14.00–17.30 | Session 4 |
| | **PHARMACOGENETICS** |
| | Chairmen: H.F. Woods (Sheffield/UK) |
| | W. Forth (München/FRG) |
| | W. Kalow (Toronto/Canada) |
| | Development and Significance of Pharmacogenetics |
| | D.S. Davies (London/UK) |
| | Polymorphism in the Cytochrome P-450 Enzyme System |
| 15.30–16.00 | Coffee Break |
| | L. Bertilsson (Huddinge/Sweden) |
| | The Pharmacokinetic Consequence of Pharmacogenetics |
| | M.S. Lennard (Sheffiel/UK) |
| | The Metabolism and Action of Beta-Adrenoceptor Antagonists in Relation of Oxidation Phenotype |
| | U.A. Meyer (Basel/Switzerland) |
| | The Importance of Pharmacogenetics in Clinical Medicine |

## Room A

FRIDAY, MARCH 9, 1984

9.00-12.30 Session 5

**IMMUNOGENETICS**

Chairmen: J.-P. Colombo (Bern/Switzerland)
G. Riethmüller (München/FRG)

A. Svejgaard (København/Denmark)
HLA and Disease

J. Hors (Paris/France)
The HLA-System and Cancer

10.30-11.00 Coffee Break

G.O.'Neill (München/FRG)
Genetics of MHC-linked Complement Components

E. Albert (München/FRG)
Hemochromatosis and HLA Association

M.S. Hershfield (Durham/USA)
Immunodeficiency Diseases Associated with Inborn Erros of Purine Metabolism

Lunch

---

14.00-17.00 Session 6

**NUTRITION AND GENETIC DISEASE**

Chairmen: H. Bickel (Heidelberg/FRG)
G. Wolfram (München/FRG)

Ph.B. Acosta (Tallahassee/USA)
Nutrition Support of Maternal Hyperphenylalaninemia

R. Gitzelmann (Zürich/Switzerland)
Galactosemia: How does Longterm Treatment Change the Outcome

15.30 - 16.00 Coffee Break

J. Frézal, J.M. Saudubray, H. Ogier, A. Munnich,
C. Charpentier (Paris/France)
Nutritional Management of Oculo-Cutaneous Tyrosinosis and of Multiple Carboxylase Defects

# Main Speakers

Prof. Dr. E. Albert
Kinderpoliklinik
Pettenkoferstraße 8a
8000 München 2

Prof. Dr. P. B. Acosta
Florida State University
College of Home Economics
Department of Nutrition and
Food Science
Tallahassee
Florida 3 23 06
USA

Dr. U. Beisiegel
Institut für Humangenetik
der Universität Marburg
Bahnhofstraße 7a
3550 Marburg

Prof. Dr. L. Bertilsson
Department of Clinical Pharmacology
Huddinge University Hospital
141 86 Huddinge
Sweden

Prof. Dr. D. S. Davies
University London
Royal Postgraduate Medical School
Hammersmith Hospital
Ducane Road
London W12 OHS
Great Britain

Prof. Dr. V. Figura
Physiologisch-Chemisches Institut
der Westfälischen Wilhelm-Universität
Waldeyerstraße 15
4400 Münster

Prof. Dr. J. Frézal
Clinique de Génétique Médicale
Hopital des Enfants Malades
149, Rue de Sévres
75730 Paris Cedex 15
France

Prof. Dr. R. Gitzelmann
Stoffwechselabteilung der
Universitäts-Kinderklinik
Steinwiesstraße 75
8032 Zürich
Schweiz

M.S. Hershfield, M.D.
Associate Professor of Medicine
Division of Metabolism
Endocrinology and Genetics
Duke University Medical Center
Durham
27710 North Carolina
USA

Prof. Dr. W. Hörz
Institut für Physiologische Chemie
Physikalische Biochemie und Zellbiologie
Goethestraße 33
8000 München 2

Dr. Jacques Hors
c/o Prof. Dausset
INSERM r 93, Centre Hayem
Hospital St. Louis
2, Place D Fournier
75475 Paris, Cedex 10
France

Prof. W. Kalow
Department of Pharmacology
Medical Science Building
University of Toronto
Toronto
Canada M5 S1A8

Dr. M.S. Lennard
University of Sheffield
Department of Therapeutics
Hallamshire Hospital
Glossop Road
Sheffield S10 2 Jf
UK

Prof. Dr. U. A. Meyer
Biozentrum der Universität Basel
Abteilung Pharmakologie
Klingelbergstraße 70
4056 Basel
Schweiz

Prof. Dr. A. W. Nienhuis
National Institut of Health
Bethesda Maryland
USA

Dr. Geoffrey O'Neill
c/o Institut für Immunologie
der Universität München
Schillerstraße 42
8000 München 2

Prof. Dr. M. F. Niermeijer
Department of Clinical Genetics
Erasmus University
Postbus 17 38
3000 DR Rotterdam

Prof. Dr. M. F. Perutz
Medical Research Council
Laboratory of Molecular Biology
Cambridge
Great Britain

Prof. H. Ropers
Institut für Humangenetik
Albertstraße 11
7800 Freiburg

Prof. Dr. K. Sandhoff
Institut für Organische Chemie und
Biochemie
Gerhard-Domagk-Straße 1
5300 Bonn 1

Dr. Arne Svejgaard
Tissue Typing Laboratory
Ringhospitalet
University Hospital
Blegdamsvej 9
2100 Kopenhavn
Danmark

Dr. G. Utermann
Institut für Humangenetik
der Universität Marburg
Bahnhofstraße 7 a
3550 Marburg

Prof. Dr. F. Vogel
Institut für Antropologie
und Humangenetik
Postfach
6900 Heidelberg

Prof. Dr. R. Williamson
Biochemistry Department
St. Mary's Hospital
Medical School
University of London
London W 2
Great Britain

## **Short Communications,** Room B

WEDNESDAY, MARCH 7, 1984

MOLECULAR MECHANISMS
Chairmen: W. Gutensohn (München/FRG)

9.00 E.U. Griese, E. Kohne, E. Kleihauer, J. Horst (Ulm)
Analysis of the α-Globin Gene Region in German Families with α-Thalassemia Syndromes

9.15 R. Oehme, E. Kohne, E. Kleihauer, J. Horst (Ulm)
Identification of Defective Human Globin Genes by Direct and Indirect DNA Analysis

9.30 E.F. Stange, J.M. Dietschy (Ulm/Dallas)
Cholesterol Synthesis and Low Density Lipoprotein Uptake are Regulated Independently in Rat Small Intestinal Epithelium

9.45 H.A. Dresel, U. Frees, D.P. Via, J. Augustin, M. Stöhr (Heidelberg/Houston)
Characterization of Low Density Lipoprotein Binding to White Blood Cells of Normals and Familial Hypercholesterolemia by Flow Cytometry

10.00 A. J. Wieczorek, N. Zöllner (München)
Membrane-Bound Enzymes in Familial Hypercholesterolemia Studied in Human Skin Fibroblasts

10.15 I. Hillmar, N. Zöllner (München)
Effects of Platelet-Activating Factor on cAMP-Concentration in Hepatocytes and Platelets are Correlated with Platelet Aggregation

10.30 Coffee Break

11.00 A. Roscher, F. Paltauf,
B. Molzer, I. Mutz, H. Bernheimer, B. Hadorn (Graz)
Diagnosis of Zellweger Syndrome by Radioassay of Plasmalogen-Biosynthesis in Cultured Fibroblasts

11.15 F. Kase, I.B. Björkhem, P. Hågå, J.I. Pedersen (Oslo/Stockholm)
Impaired Biosynthesis of Cholic Acid in a Patient with Zellweger Cerebro-Hepato-Renal Syndrome

11.30 G.E.J. Staal, G. Jansen, D. Roos (Utrecht/Amsterdam)
Pyruvate Kinase and the "High ATP" Syndrome

11.45 T. Deufel, D. Pongratz, G. Hübner, O.H. Wieland (München)
Adult-Onset Myopathies in Glycogenoses: Biochemical and Morphological Findings

12.00 I. Paetzke, M. Bürger, T. Deufel, J. Müller-Höcker, G. Hübner, D. Pongratz, O.H. Wieland (München/Giessen)
Cytochrome-c-Oxidase Deficiency in Two Siblings with Congenital Lactic Acidemia, Disturbances of Amino acid Metabolism, and Diffuse Mitochondrial Myopathy

12.15 J. Müller-Höcker, D. Pongratz, G. Hübner (München)
Defective Mitochondrial Function in the Skeletal Muscle of Patients with Progressive External Ophthalmoplegia

Lunch

# Abstracts

## ANALYSIS OF THE α-GLOBIN GENE REGION IN GERMAN FAMILIES WITH α-THALASSEMIA SYNDROMES

Griese[1], E.-U., Kohne[2], E., Kleihauer[2], E. Horst[1], J.

Abteilung Humangenetik[1] and Pädiatrie II[2], Universität Ulm, 7900 Ulm, FRG.

The α-thalassemia (thal) syndromes are inherited anemias characterized by a decrease in or absence of synthesis of α-globin chains, resulting in four clinical states of increasing severity: α-thal-2, α-thal-1, Hb H disease and hydrops fetalis Hb Bart's syndrome. α-globin gene deletion is the predominant underlaying molecular defect in Asian, Black and Mediterranean populations. Non-deletion forms have been detected with much lower overall frequency and mainly in patients of Mediterranean origin. Since so far nothing was known about the α-globin gene defect in central European derived α-thal patients, DNA mapping experiments were performed of the chromosomal DNA from two unrelated German families with α-thal affected members. The DNA pattern obtained indicated loss of α-globin genes in all α-thal affected individuals. In α-thal-1 individuals both α-genes were deleted from one chromosome (- -/αα). In α-thal-2 (- /αα) and Hb H (- -/-α) individuals the chromosomes showing loss of one α-gene were characterized by the so-called rightward deletion of a 3.7 kb DNA fragment in the α-globin gene cluster.

## IDENTIFICATION OF DEFECTIVE HUMAN GLOBIN GENES BY DIRECT AND INDIRECT DNA ANALYSIS

Oehme[1], R., Kohne[2], E., Kleihauer[2], E. Horst[1], J.

Abteilung Humangenetik[1] and Pädiatrie II[2], Universität Ulm, 7900 Ulm, FRG.

Chromosomal DNA of patients with Hb M Milwaukee, Hb Köln and Hb Presbyterian was analysed by DNA restriction methods. The direct detection of the mutant

Hb M Milwaukee ß-globin gene in three generations of an afflicted family could be achieved by endonuclease Sst I digestion. Blot hybridization using the ß-globin probe revealed three fragments of 15.5, 9.0 and 6.5 Kb, a pattern found by us to be diagnostic for the heterozygous state of Hb M Milwaukee in preliminary studies (Brit.J.Haematol. 54, 643, 1983). Normal controls exhibited the 15.5 Kb fragment only. To identify the mutant Hb Köln and Hb Presbyterian ß-globin genes seven restriction sites (Hinc II$\varepsilon$, Hind III$^{G}\gamma$ , Hind III$^{A}\gamma$, Hinc II$\psi$ß, Hinc II 3'$\psi$ß, Ava IIß, Bam HIß) were analysed that have been found to be polymorphic within the ß-globin gene cluster (Antonarakis et al. Proc. Nat. Acad. Sci. USA 79, 137, 1982).
DNA blotting and hybridization with specific $\varepsilon$-. $\gamma$-. $\psi$ ß1- and ß-globin probes revealed that in the families under investigation the haplotype constellation + - - - - + + and - + - + + - + were diagnostic for the Hb Köln and Hb Presbyterian ß-globin gene carrying chromosomes respectively. Data on the frequences of chromosomal haplotype constellation of the ß-globin gene cluster in populations of central European origin are discussed.

## CHOLESTEROL SYNTHESIS AND LOW DENSITY LIPOPROTEIN UPTAKE ARE REGULATED INDEPENDENTLY IN RAT SMALL INTESTINAL EPITHELIUM

*Stange*[+], *E.F.*, *Dietschy*, *J.M.*

Department of Internal Medicine, University of Texas Health Science Center, Dallas, Texas ([+]current address: University Clinic Ulm, Department of Internal Medicine, Ulm, FRG)

We have compared the rates of low density lipoprotein (LDL) uptake and cholesterol synthesis in the rat intestine. By using a constant infusion technique, total and receptor -independent uptake was determined with homologous rat LDL (rLDL) and methylated human LDL (Me-hLDL), respectively. The absolute rates of sterel synthesis were measured with [1-$^{14}$C]-octanoate and [$^{3}$H ] water. The rates of rLDL uptake in whole gut segments were similar along the length of the small intestine, whereas the rates of sterol synthesis varied over a 5-fold range and were highest in the duodenum and distal ileum. When the mucosal epithelium was fractionated along the villus/crypt axis, both rLDL and Me-hLDL clearance by the enterocytes increased approximately 3-fold in going from the upper villus to the crypt cell fractions, in both jejunum and ileum. In both the whole gut segments and isolated cells, approximately 60% of LDL uptake was receptor-dependent. When the rates of rLDL cholesterol uptake were calculated and related to the absolute rates of sterol synthesis in the same cell fractions in vivo, both processes were found to be distributed similarly along the villus/crypt axis. Furthermore, the majority of mucosal cholesterol (64-86%) was derived from local synthesis rather than from rLDL uptake at all locations along the intestinal villus. Finally, when sterol synthesis in the epithelial cells was varied up to 7-fold by feeding cholesterol, triglyceride, cholestyramine, or surfomer, rLDL uptake was essentially unchanged. Thus, in intestinal epithelial cells in vivo, the rate of LDL uptake was constant under circumstances in which changing needs for cellular cholesterol were met by changes in the rates of sterol synthesis.

## CHARACTERIZATION OF LOW DENSITY LIPOPROTEIN BINDING TO WHITE BLOOD CELLS OF NORMALS AND FAMILIAL HYPERCHOLESTEROLEMIA BY FLOW CYTOMETRY

*Dresel, H.A.*[+], *Frees, U.*[+], *Via, D.P.*[*], *Augustin, J.*[+], *Stöhr, M.*[++],

[+]Medizinische Klinik der Universität Heidelberg
Bergheimer Str. 58, D-6900 Heidelberg, FRG

[*]Department of Medicine, Baylor College of Medicine
6565 Fannin A-601, Houston/Texas 77030, USA

[++]Inst.f. Experimentelle Pathologie
Deutsches Krebsforschungszentrum, D-6900 Heidelberg, FRG

Patients with familial hypercholesterolemia do not catabolize circulatory low density lipoprotein (LDL) effieciently because their cells have a genetic deficiency in surface LDL receptors that normally mediate the uptake of LDL by cells. Cells swollen with cholesterol esters are found in the patient' atheromatic lesions of the arterial wall and are called foam cells. Foam cells are believed to have a macorphage origin.

Chemically modified LDL derived by acetylation is degraded rapidly by macrophages via an "acetyl-LDL receptor" mediated pathway which differs from the classical LDL receptor pathway. Incubation of macrophages in vitro leads to generation of cells with the general appearance of foam cells. It is therefore hypothesized that the acetyl-LDL receptor on monocyte/macrophage like cells might have importance in the pathogenesis of atherosclerosis.

In the experiments we report the binding of LDL and acetyl-LDL labelled with fluorescent cholesterol ester by freshly isolated mononuclear leukocytes from normals and patients with familial hypercholesterolemia. Combining light scattering and fluorescence parameters of cells it was possible to characterize low density lipoprotein binding to leukocytes and selected subpopulations of white blood cells by flow cytometry.

## MEMBRANE-BOUND ENZYMES IN FAMILIAL HYPERCHOLESTEROLEMIA, STUDIED IN HUMAN SKIN FIBROBLASTS

*Wieczorek, A.J., Zöllner, N.*

Medizinische Poliklinik, D-8000 Munich 2, Pettenkoferstraße 8a, FRG

Most of the enzymes of synthesis are membrane-bound including Golgi enzymes and enzymes of the endoplasmatic reticulum. These enzymes require an undisturbed lipid environment for controlled activity. The best model for studying these enzymes in a disturbed lipid environment is familial hypercholesterolemia with its low cholesterol ester content in the membranes.

We chose two enzymes which are of special interest in familial hypercholesterolemia: ceramide-glucosyltransferase and glucuronyltransferase.

The first is a key enzyme in glycosphingolipid synthesis which was found increased in familial hypercholesterolemia. The second is a key enzyme in the synthesis of glycosaminoglycans which exhibit a high affinity for low-density lipoprotein.

Ceramide-glucosyltransferase was assayed by addition of $^{14}C$ ceramide to isolated Golgi fraction of healthy (n = 8) and homozygous familial hypercholesterolemic skin fibroblasts (n = 6). Glucosyl ceramide, the reaction product, was isolated by thin layer chromatography (silica gel, chloroform/methanol/water, 65:25:4). Glucuronyltransferase was assayed by incorporation of UDP- $^{14}C$ glucuronic acid into endogeneous microsomal acceptors.

The activities of both membrane-bound enzymes were found increased in familial hypercholesterolemia (ceramide-glucosyltransferase $2.3 \pm 0.2$ pmol/mg cell protein x min (controls $0.8 \pm 0.1$ pmol/mg x min), glucuronyltransferase 4.8 pmol/mg x min, SD 0.3 (controls $1.3 \pm 0.1$ pmol/mg x min)).

The results can provide an explanation for hitherto not understood phenomena in familial hypercholesterolemia.

EFFECTS OF PLATELET-ACTIVATING FACTOR ON cAMP-CONCENTRATION IN HEPATOCYTES AND PLATELETS IS CORRELATED WITH PLATELET AGGREGATION

*Hillmar, I., Zöllner, N.*

Forschergruppe Ernährung an der Medizinischen Poliklinik der Universität München, Schillerstr. 42, 8 München 2, W.-Germany

1-O-Alkyl-2-acetoyl-sn-glycero-3-phosphocholine (PAF) acts on cAMP-concentrations in hepatocyte suspensions and in human platelets. The hepatocyte is detected as target cell for PAF. The cAMP-decreasing effect is correlated with aggregatory potency in platelets and molecular mechanisms of PAF-action are discussed.

PAF and a analogue with a mixture of saturated and unsaturated alkyl moities (U-PAF) lower cAMP-concentrations in hepatocytes at $10^{-6}$M by 51 % and 53 %. Activity is observed between $10^{-6}$M and $10^{-12}$M. The thio compound, with the thio group instead of an ether linkage acts in the same range in hepatocytes.

PAF, U-PAF and Thio-PAF ($10^{-4}$M) decrease cAMP-content in platelets by 37 %, 31 % and 25 % during 30 minutes incubation. When cAMP-concentrations are elevated by 2 µg/ml prostaglandin $E_1$ in hepatocytes, PAF-induced suppression of cAMP is abolished.

Alterations in cAMP are correlated with the aggregatory potency of the three analogue inplatelets, compared between $10^{-4}$M and $10^{-8}$M. PAF-mediated aggregation is independent of ADP-release and formation of arachidonic acid products. Preliminary experiments demonstrate binding of $^{3}$H-PAF on isolated rat hepatocytes.

# DIAGNOSIS OF ZELLWEGER SYNDROME BY RADIOASSAY OF PLASMALOGEN-BIOSYNTHESIS IN CULTURED FIBROBLASTS

*Roscher, A., Paltauf, F., Molzer, B., Mutz, I., Bernheimer, H., Hadorn, B.*

Department of Paediatrics, University of Graz, Auenbruggerplatz, A-8036 Graz, Austria

The Zellweger syndrome (ZS) is a rare autosomal recessive disorder with abnormalities in several organ systems (cerebro-hepato-renal syndrome). On a subcellular level a deficiency of peroxisomes in liver and kidney has been recognized. Since the initial steps of 1-o-(1-alkenyl) glycerolipid (plasmalogen)-biosynthesis proceed in peroxisomes this pathway was studied in fibroblasts of affected patients.

Phospholipid (PL) analysis revealed a marked deficiency of plasmalogens in ZS fibroblasts (ZS : 4.0 $\pm$ 1.1 % of total PL, N : 13.8 $\pm$ 1.4 %). No difference in the relative distribution of other PL was found. This defect was further characterized by incubating intact fibroblasts for various periods of time with ($^{14}C$) hexadecanol and ($^{3}H$) hexadecylglycerol. ($^{14}C$) hexadecanol-incorporation into plasmalogens was almost abolished in ZS fibroblasts (0.6 $\pm$ 0.3 %) as compared to controls (15.0 $\pm$ 4.0 % of total incorporated).

($^{3}H$) hexadecylglycerol, however, was utilized to a similar extent by both genotypes. The results indicate that plasmalogen-biosynthesis in ZS is altered at the level of the alkyldihydroxyacetonphosphate-synthesis. This finding appears to be specific for ZS since normal ether-lipid biosynthesis was found in fibroblasts of patients with neuronal ceroidlipofuscinosis (NCLF) and in adrenoleucodystrophy (ALD). In contrast, ZS and ALD fibroblasts both exhibited augmented levels of $C_{26}$ : 0 very long chain fatty acids.

Incubation of intact cells with radiolabelled precursors of ether-lipid biosynthesis and subsequent radioassay of $^{3}H/^{14}C$ ratios in plasmalogens might provide a highly sensitive and specific test for the (prenatal) diagnosis of ZS.

## IMPAIRED BIOSYNTHESIS OF CHOLIC ACID IN A PATIENT WITH ZELLWEGER CEREBRO-HEPATO-RENAL SYNDROME

*Kase*[1], F., *Björkhem*[2], I., *Hågå*[3], P., *Pedersen*[1], J.I.

1) Inst. for Nutrition Research, University of Oslo, Norway
2) Dep. of Clin. Chem., Huddinge Hospital, Karolinska Institutet, Stockholm, Sweden
3) Dep. of Pediatrics, Ulleval Hospital, Oslo, Norway

Zellweger syndrome is an autosomal recessive disorder characterized by impaired biosynthesis of bile acids and absence of liver peroxisomes.

$3\alpha$, $7\alpha$, $12\alpha$-Trihydroxy-5ß-cholestanoic acid (THCA) is detected in increased amounts in the serum and bile indicating a reduced capacity of oxidative cleavage of the $C_{27}$-steroid side chain. To test this hypothesis 10µCi $[^3H]$-5ß-cholestane-$3\alpha$, $7\alpha$, $12\alpha$-triol was given intravenously to a patient with Zellweger syndrome. x) Serum and bile were analyzed for labelled products. After 24 hours two main tritiated products in serum were separated on HPLC and identified on GC - MS as THCA and the other was a product with oxidation of one of the C-atoms in the side chain of THCA. Cholic acid was a minor product. No trace of the given triol was recovered. In duodenal aspirate THCA dominated 3 hours after infusion and declined slowly. The formation of cholic acid increased to 15 % of given triol 24 hours after infusion when it levelled off.

The results support the conclusion that in Zellweger syndrome there is an incomplete block in the conversion of THCA to cholic acid, probably at the level of the liver peroxisomes.

x) The ethical aspects of the present study was approved by the ethical board of the Norwegian Council for Science and Humanities.

## PYRUVATE KINASE AND THE "HIGH ATP" SYNDROME

*Staal*[1], G.E.J., *Jansen*[1], G., *Roos*[2], D.

1) Department of Hematology, Division of Medical Enzymology, Academic Hospital Utrecht, 3500 CG Utrecht, The Netherlands
2) Central Laboratory of the Netherlands Red cross Blood Transfusion Service, Amsterdam, The Netherlands

Pyruvate kinase (ATP; pyruvate phosphotransferase, EC 2.7.1.40) catalyzes the conversion of phosphoenolpyruvate to pyruvate with the generation of ATP. Pyruvate kinase deficiency results in a diminished capacity to regenerate ATP and the content of 2,3-DPG may be increased occasionally. A hereditary increase of red cell ATP has been described only in a few cases. We report on an abnormality which is characterized by high erythrocyte ATP (180 to 200 percent of the normal value), increased pyruvate kinase activity (about twice the normal level) and decreased 2,3-DPG content. Other glycolytic enzymes are in the normal range. The mode of inheritance is autosomal dominant. The marked increase in pyruvate kinase activity is believed to be responsible for the high ATP. Characterization of pyruvate kinase showed that the high pyruvate kinase activity is due to a shift in the R T equilibrium to the R-state: increased affinity for the substrate phosphoenolpyruvate, decreased inhibition by ATP, decreased influence of fructose-1,6-$P_2$. The $K_m$ for ADP, thermostability, pH optimum, electrophoresis and immunological specific activity are normal.

## ADULT-ONSET MYOPATHIES IN GLYCOGENOSES: BIOCHEMICAL AND MORPHOLOGICAL FINDINGS

*Deufel*[1], T., *Pongratz*[2], D., *Hübner*[3], G., *Wieland*[1], O.H.

Inst. f. Klin.Chemie, Krankenhaus München-Schwabing (1), Friedr.-Baur-Inst., Med.Klinik Innenstadt (2) and Pathologisches Inst. (3) der Univers.,Munich,FRG.

Findings in adult forms of glycogenoses differ considerably from the usual pattern. In this study, morphological and biochemical data on patients with adult-onset acid maltase deficiency (AMD) and myophosphorylase deficiency

(MPD) are presented.
In two of three cases of adult-onset AMD, slowly progressive muscular weakness beginning beyond the fourth decade was the leading symptom. Muscle morphology in these cases showed glycogen filled vacuoles in single fibers, whereas large areas of tissue seemed unaffected. In a third case, however, the clinical symptoms suggested neurogenic muscular atrophy, and muscle biopsy showed severe tissue degeneration, but also in some fibers glycogen filled vacuoles, some of them surrounded by membranes, as seen in AMD. Biochemical measurements showed decreased acid maltase, but normal glycogen in all three cases. Lysosomal N-acetyl-glucosaminidase was elevated in the latter, but normal in the two myopathic cases.
In two patients with MPD onset of symptoms was in the fifth decade of live with muscular weakness, no contractures were oberserved. Muscle biopsies showed diffuse subsarcolemmal accumulation of glycogen, consistent with MPD. On biochemical examination phosphorylase was absent, glycogen was found to be increased appr. 2folds. SDS electrophoresis of soluble muscle proteins demonstrated absence of the phosporylase band ($M_r$ = 92 000), as in juvenile cases investigated before, in one case, but an atypical band ($M_r$ = 95 000) in the other.
Theses heterogeneous findings indicate that clinical variations cannot be explained by presence of a distinct subtype in adult-onset MPD.

## CYTOCHROME-c-OXIDASE DEFICIENCY IN TWO SIBLINGS WITH CONGENITAL LACTIC ACIDEMIA, DISTURBANCES OF AMINOACID METABOLISM, AND DIFFUSE MITOCHONDRIAL MYOPATHY

*Paetzke[1], I., Bürger[2], M., Deufel[1], T., Müller-Höcker[3], J., Hübner[3], G., Pongratz[4], D., Wieland[1], O.H.,*

Inst.f.Klin.Chem.Krankenhs.München-Schwabing (1), Zentr. f. Kinderheilkunde, Univ.Giessen (2), Patholog.Inst.Universität München (3) and Friedr.-Baur-Inst., Med.Klinik Innenstadt, Univers.München (4), Munich, FRG.

Two siblings are described suffering from congenital lactic acidemia and disturbances in aminoacid metabolism. The elder child died in the age of four weeks. Muscle biopsy obtained before death showed cytochrome-c-oxidase activity to be less than 10 % of the normal mean, when based on glutamatedehydrogenase as a mitochondrial marker. A disorder of muscle mitochondria was suggested by morphological and electron microscopical findings, showing increased and partially enlarged mitochondria. The cytochemical-ultrastructural cytochrome-c-oxidase

reaction was extremely faint.
In the younger child disturbances of aminoacid metabolism were diagnosed in amniotic fluid before birth. Muscle biopsy gave nearly identical changes as found in the elder child. Increased and morphologically abnormal mitochondria are recognized by light and elctron microscopy Cytochrome-c-oxidase activity was decreased, but to a lesser degree than in the sib. Muscle biopsies of both parents did not show biochemical abnormalities, but morphological examination showed focal abnormalities of mitochondria. In conclusion, the infantile mitochondrial myopathy with congenital lactic acidemia is supposed to be due to cytochrome-c-oxidase defciency, with probable autosomal recessive inheritance.

## DEFECTIVE MITOCHONDRIAL FUNCTION IN THE SKELETAL MUSCEL OF PATIENTS WITH PROGRESSIVE EXTERNAL OPHTHALMOPLEGIA

*Müller-Höcker, J., Pongratz, D., Hübner, G.,*

Pathologsiches Institut und Med. Klinik Innenstadt der Universität, 8000 München 2, Thalkirchnerstr. 36

Progressive external ophthalmoplegia (PEO) is a complex disorder with multiorgan involvement. External ocular and skeletal muscles are regularly affected. In addition retinal, cerebral and cardiac maifestations are known to occur, among other symptoms. The changes in skeletal muscle are best described as mitochondrial myopathy with accumulation of enlarged, structurally abnormal mitochondria in single fibres, and with increased storage or lipid. However, biochemical studies so far have failed to reveal any consistent of specific abnormalities. We therefore undertook an enzyme histochemical, immunocytochemical and fine structural study in order to get deeper insigth into mytochondrial function using skeletal muscle biopsies of 8 patients with PEO.
Combined. light and electron microscopic demonstration of cytochrome-c-oxidase revealed as constant finding variable amounts of fibres with complete absence of enzyme acitivity,irrespective of the concomitant structural alterations, i.e. the enzyme defect was present in normal appearing fibres as well as in those with accumulation of abnormal mitochondria. However, some fibres had abnormal mitochondria without any deficiency of the enzyme. Immunocytochemistry of cytochrome-c-oxidase showed very weak, or no reaction in fibres with the enzyme defect. Cytochemical investigation of mitochondrial ATPase demonstrated acti-

vation of the ATP-synthesising enzyme in single fibres prior to stimulation by an uncoupler, this indicating loosely coupled oxidative phosphorylation, respectively damage to the inner mitochondrial membrane (to which the respiratory chain is linked). In some fibres the enzyme activity was completely absent. - The results are consistent with a gradually developing mitochondrial damage leading to defective function of the respiratory chain in single skeletal fibres of patients with PEO. Immunocytochemistry of cytochrome-c-oxidase shows that the enzyme defect is based on a highly diminished enzyme content. Therefore loss of enzyme from the inner mitochondrial membrane, perhaps because of a membrane defect, increased turnover, decreased and/or faulty synthesis of the enzyme itself have to be considered. Concerning the defective base of the disease, the question arises whether the defective mitochondrial function in PEO is due to derangements of nuclear and/or mitochondrial DNA coding for mitochondrial proteins.

## **Short Communications,** Room B

WEDNESDAY, MARCH 7, 1984

INBORN ERRORS OF THE ADULT
Chairmen: G. Paumgartner (München/FRG)

| | |
|---|---|
| 14.00 | K. Tada, K. Narisawa, Y. Igarashi (Sendai)<br>Genetic Heterogeneity of Glycogen Storage Disease Type I B between Infantile Cases and Adult Cases |
| 14.15 | A. Kohlschütter, H. H. Goebel (Hamburg/Mainz)<br>Diagnosis of Pompe Disease (Glycogenosis II) by Morphologic and Enzymatic Analysis of Blood Lymphocytes |
| 14.30 | D. Alexander, G. Dudin, M. Deeb, F. Talj, V.D. Kaloustian (Beirut)<br>Biochemical Studies on Five Related Lebanese Individuals with High Plasma Lysosomal Enzymes |
| 14.45 | K. Ullrich, E.M. Brouwer-Kelder, A.W. Schram, J.M. Tager, D. von Bassewitz, R. Korinthenberg, H. Gröbe, K. von Figura (Münster/Amsterdam)<br>-Galactosidase Deficiency: Variant of Fabry's Disease with Mild Clinical Expression and Pseudodeficiency of Serum $\alpha$-Galactosidase |
| 15.00 | E. Paschke, H. Kresse (Graz/Münster)<br>Increased Activity of Partially Purified Urinary $G_{M1}$ ß-Galactosidase from an Adult Morquio B-Patient in the Presence of $G_{M1}$-Activator Protein |
| 15.15 | G. Boers, B. Fowler, J. Trijbels, A. Smals, P. Kloppenborg (Nijmegen /Manchester)<br>Heterozygosity for Homocystinuria as a Risk Factor of Premature Arteriosclerosis |
| 15.30 | Coffee Braek |

16.00 E. Harms, G. Gallasch (Heidelberg)
Hyperornithinemia with Gyrate Atrophy of the Choroid and Retina

16.15 D.Overkamp, B.Jakober,E.Weidle, H.J.Thiel, M.Eggstein (Tübingen)
Richner Hanhart Syndrome along with Morbus Wilson

16.30 W.Lehnert, H.Niederhoff (Freiburg)
2-Methylacetoacetyl-CoA Thiolase Deficiency.
In Vitro Studies with Deuterated Metabolites in Three Patients

16.45 L.Konarska, L. Tomaszewski (Warsaw)
Sensitive, Quantitative, Simple Screening Test for Arginase Deficiency

17.00 R.W.E. Watts, P. Purkiss, N. Veall (Harrow)
Oxalate Dynamics in Primary Hyperoxaluria and Renal Failure

17.15 H.F.M. Busch, H.R. Scholte, I.E.M. Luyt-Houwen, W.F.M. Arts (Rotterdam)
A Mitochondrial Myopathy with a Deficiency of NADH-CoQ Reductase Activity in a Mother and Son

17.30 H.R. Scholte, M. de Visser, R.B.H. Schutgens, I.E.M. Luyt-Houwen (Rotterdam/Amsterdam)
A Riboflavin-Responsive Patient with Glutaric Aciduria Type II and Her Three Asymptomatic Sisters, All with a Defective Mitochondrial Beta Oxidation in Muscle & Fibroblasts and Severe Systemic Carnitine Deficiency

# GENETIC HETEROGENEITY OF GLYCOGEN STORAGE DISEASE TYPE IB BETWEEN INFANTILE CASES AND ADULT CASES

*Tada, K., Narisawa, K., Igarashi, Y.*

Department of Pediatrics, Tohoku University Medical School, Sendai, Japan

In 1978, we reported that a basic defect in GSD type 1b was located in the glucose-6-phosphate (G6P) transport system of the microsomal membrane, based on the findings that the glucose-6-phosphatase activity was highly latent in the fresh liver homogenate (1,2).
In infantile cases of GSD type 1b, the patients show early onset of clinical symptoms, rapid development of hypoglycemia, neutropenia and frequent infections. On the other hand, adult cases of type 1b, the patients have mild clinical symptoms and did not show neurotropenia and episodes of recurrent infections. In order to elucidate the difference between these two clinical types, the activity of G6P translocase was investigated, using biopsied liver specimens.
The activity of G6P translocase was undetectable in infantile case, whereas the residual activity (about 8% of the normal) was found in an adult case. These findings indicate that the clinical severitiy of this disorder depends on the level of the residual activity of the G6P translocase. A kinetic study of the residual G6P translocase in the adult patient showed 16 times higher Km for G6P as compared with that of controls, suggesting the structual gene mutation.

References:

1. Narisawa, K., Igarashi, Y., Otomo, H. and Tada,K.: Biochem. Biophsy. Res. Comm., 83:1360 /1979)
2. Igarashi, Y., Otomo, H.,Narisawa, K. and Tada, K.: J. Inherit. Metab. Dis., 2:45 (1979)

# DIAGNOSIS OF POMPE DISEASE (GLYCOGENOSIS II) BY MORPHOLOGIC AND ENZYMATIC ANALYSIS OF BLOOD LYMPHOCYTES

Kohlschütter[1], A., Goebel[2], H.H.

[1]Dept. of Pediatrics, Hamburg University, D-2000 Hamburg, 20
[2]Dept. of Neuropathology, Mainz University, D-6500 Mainz

The definitive diagnosis of a lysosomal storage disorder depends on the demonstration of both the accumulated specific metabolite and the defective enzymatic degradation of this metabolite. In Pompe disease this is usually accomplished by the study of muscle tissue, where an accumulation of glycogen and a deficient lysosomal acid glucosidase is found. The use of mixed blood leucocytes or of urine for the enzymatic diagnosis of Pompe disease is unreliable because of the interference of non-lysosomal glucosidases (2).
Since isolated lymphocytes are a valuable object for ultrastructural studies in a suspected storage disorder (1), we have used lymphocytes prepared from small amounts of blood for both electron microscopic and enzymatic analysis in several cases of the adult (muscular) and the infantile (generalized) variety of Pompe disease. Glycogen accumulation in lymphocyte inclusions was clearly recognizable by its unique granular appearance. -glucosidase activity in homogenates from isolated lymphocytes was measured in the pH range from 3 to 7. Normal lymphocytes had a distinct pH optimum in the acid and a second one in the neutral range. All cases of Pompe disease showed an unquestionable absence of the acid component. Parents of infantile cases had about half normal activities of this compound.
In Pompe disease, isolated blood lymphocytes show the excess accumulation of glycogen and an enzymatic pattern analogous to that of muscle tissue. Biopsies may be avoided.

References:

1) Ikeda, K. et al., Eur. J. Pediatr. 138:179-185 (1982)
2) Pilz, H. et al., J. Clin. Chem. Clin. Biochem. 15:705-708 (1977)

BIOCHEMICAL STUDIES ON FIVE RELATED LEBANESE INDIVIDUALS WITH HIGH PLASMA LYSOSOMAL ENZYMES

*Alexander, D., Dudin, G., Deeb, M., Talj, F., Vazken Der Kaloustian*

National Unit of Human Genetics, American University of Beirut Medical Center, Beirut, Lebanon.

A Lebanese family has been found in which 5 clinically normal relatives in 3 generations have plasma levels of at least 7 lysosomal enzymes up to 94x control values, whilst their urine and CSF enzyme values are normal. The pattern and extent of plasma lysosomal enzyme elevation is similar to that observed in I-cell disease. Plasma $\alpha$-mannosidase has been found to have physicochemical properties distinct from control, and fibroblasts from one of the 5 relatives secreted 2-7 control levels of lysosomal enzymes into cell culture media (submitted for publication). Further studies have now been carried out to characterize the oligosaccharide moieties of plasma enzymes. Seven lysosomal hydrolases were separated on a column of Concanavalin A-Sepharose 4B (Con A) by eluting with 10 mM $\alpha$-methylglucoside (MG) and 100 mM $\alpha$-methylmannoside (MM). The abnormally elevated enzymes bound strongly to Con A, and there was a marked reduction in the % of unbound lysosomal enzymes as compared to those in control plasma e.g. 19% of $\alpha$-fucosidase and 6.4 % of hexosaminidase B (hex B) remained unbound in control plasma, but 0.5 % of both in the abnormal plasma. $\alpha$-fucosidase, hex B and ß-glucuronidase were isolated form the peaks eluted from the Con A column and treated with endoglycosidase H (endo H) before re-running on Con A. After endo H treatment, 42 % of the hex B and 64 % of the $\alpha$-fucosidase from the MG eluted peak no longer bound to Con A, whilst 16 % of the hex B but none of the $\alpha$-fucosidase or ß-glucuronidase from the MM peak were unbound. The strong binding of elevated lysosomal enzymes to Con A, together with their partial sensitivity to endo H, suggests the presence of 'high mannose'oligosaccharides on the abnormally elevated enzymes. This is in contrast to extracellular enzymes in I-cell disease in which oligosaccharides are processed to the 'complex type' (Sly WS & Fischer HD, J. Cell Biochem. 18: 67-85, 1982). When eluted from a QAE-Sephadex column, abnormal plasma hex B eluted in a position suggesting a less negative net charge compared to control plasma hex B. ß-glucuronidase from abnormal plasma was not taken up into ß-glucuronidase-deficient fibroblasts. The evidence suggests that these 5 individuals are heterozygous for an abnormal allele resulting in high accumulation of plasma lysosomal enzymes bearing oligosaccharides of the 'high mannose' rather than 'complex type', but lacking phosphomannose moieties. The mutation could be expressed in oligosaccharide synthsis or processing, or in the mannose-6-phosphate receptor.

Supported by the Lebanese National Council for Scientific Research.

## α-GALACTOSIDASE DEFICIENCY: VARIANT OF FABRY DISEASE WITH MILD CLINICAL EXPRESSION AND PSEUDODEFICIENCY OF SERUM α-GALACTOSIDASE

*Ullrich, K., Brouwer-Kelder[+], E.M., Schram[+], A.W., Tager[+], J.M., von Bassewitz[+++], D., Korinthenberg, R., Gröbe, H., von Figura, K.*

Kinderklinik, Physiolog.-Chemisches** und Pathologisches Institut***, Münster, FRG; jansen Institute*, Amsterdam, The Netherlands

Fabry disease was diagnosed in a 28 year old man with the only clinical features of cornea verticillata and tortuous conjunctival vessels. ECG, echocard, EEG, NCV and routine leboratory data were normal. Though no cutaneous maifestation of the disease was present, the typical lysosomal storage material was found in perivascular cells by electronmicroscopical examination of a skin biopsy. After prolonged wear of contact lenses, regression of cornea verticillata appeared. The deficiency ofα-galactosidase in fibroblasts was as profound as in patients with the calssical form of the disease (5 % of that of controls). In contrast to the classical form acitivites in the heterozygote to normal range were found in leucocytes, serum and urine. - Two unrelated endzymes, α-galactosidase and α-N-acetylgalactosaminidase, cleave p-nitrophenyl and 4-methylumbelliferyl-α-D-galactosides. By immunoprecipitation the relative contribution of the two enzymes to the α-galactosidase acitivity observed in serum and urine of the patient was determined and found to be normal.
In a course of a family study in a kindred with two Fabry patients α-galactosidase deficiency was detected in a healthy 40 year old male. Electronmicroscopical examination of the skin revealed no storage phenomena. Normal acitivity of α-galactosidase was found in leucocytes and fibroblasts. Over a period of 2 years the α-galactosidase activity was measured in seven samples. Deficiency of α-galactosidas towards the p-nitrophenylsubstrate was consistently found whereas on three occasions normal activity towards the 4-methylumbelliferyl-substrate was observed. This acitivity showed an abnormal pH-dependence with an additional pH-optimum at pH 3.5. Whereas in controls more than 95 % of total α- galacosidase

from pH 3-7 reacted with the antiserum against $\alpha$-galactosidase, the corresponding value for the proband was 70%. The nature of the pseudodeficiency with inacitivity towards o-nitrophenyl-$\alpha$-D-galactoside and variable activity against the 4-methylumbelliferyl-substrate in the serum remains obscure.

## INCREASED ACTIVITY OF PARTIALLY PURIFIED URINARY $G_{M1}$-ß-GALACTOSIDASE FROM AN ADULT MORQUIO B-PATIENT IN THE PRESENCE OF $G_{M1}$-ACTIVATOR PROTEIN

*Paschke*[+], *E.*, *Kresse*[++], *H.*

*Universitäts-Kinderklinik Graz, Austria and **Physiologisch-chemisches Institut der WWU, Münster, Germany

In infantile and juvenile $G_{M1}$-ganglioside deficiency of acid ß-galactosidase (ß-gal) causes symptoms of both glycolipid and keratan sulfate accummulation. Some patients with decreased ß-gal activity however show all signs of keratan sulfate but no sympomts of glycolipid storage. Urinary ß-gal from a 29-year old Morquio B-patient was studied:

The patient excreted normal amounts of enzyme protein precipitable with monospecific rabbit antiserum. In gel filtration at pH 7.0 ultrafiltrates of urine samples showed normal acitivity of the oligomeric but reduced acitivity of the monomeric enzyme form. Urinary Morquio B ß-gal paritally purified on Con A-Sepharose however eluted as a monomer at pH 7.0. It showed normal dimer formation at pH 4.0 and behaved as a $k_M$ and $V_{max}$ -mutant against pNP-ß-galactoside, ($^3$H)-keratan sulfate and a neutral ($^3$H)-pentasaccharide. Against ($^3$H)-$G_{M1}$-ganglioside a normal $k_M$ but a very low $V_{max}$ was measured in the presence of taurocholate. Thus higher activities against the oligosaccharide and keratan sulfate than against the ganglioside in the presence of taurocholate were computed. In the presence of $G_{M1}$-activator protein at tenfold increase of $G_{M1}$ ß-gal was observed yielding a twice normal ratio between pNP-ß-galactoside - and $G_{M1}$-ganglioside-ß-gal. We therefore suggest that $G_{M1}$-activator increases a distinct portion of ß-gal acitivity against $G_{M1}$ganglioside. this hould result in sufficient ganglioside degradation in vivo. Data about the $G_{M1}$-ganglioside-ß-gal from crude Morquio-B-cell h omogenates confirm this suggestion [(1)].

References:

(1): E. Paschke, H. Kresse, (1982), Biochem. Biophys. Res. Commun. 109, 568-575.

## HETEROZYGOSITY FOR HOMOCYSTINURIA AS A RISK FACTOR OF PREMATURE ARTERIOSCLERIOSIS

*Boers, G., Fowler, B.*[*]*, Trijbels, J.*[**]*, Smals, A., Kloppenborg, P.*

Department of Medicine, Division of Endocrinology, and Dept. of Pediatrics**
St. Radboud Hosp., Univ. of Nijmegen, The Netherlands.
Willink Biochemical Genetics Unit, Royal Manchester Children's Hosp., Univ. of Manchester, Great-Britain*

In homozygous homocystinuria (HOA) premature arteriosclerosis with thromboembolic events is the most serious complication. Heterozygositiy for HOA has not been reported to be associated with proneness to premature arteriosclerosis. To determine the incidence of excessive homocysteinemia after methionine (M)-loading in groups of patients suffering from premature arteriosclerosis in the absence of known risk factors, we performed a standardized M-Loading (0.1 g/kg) in: i, a group of 25 patients, under the age of 50, with occlusive cerebrovascular disease, ii, a group of 23 patients, under the age of 50, with peripheral arteriosclerosis (in ateria iliaca, renalis, or mesenterica) or recurrent thromboembolisms, iii, a group of 14 patients, under the age of 45, suffering form myocardial infarction. In all patients diabetes, hyperlipoproteinemia and hypertension were excluded. After-load serum levels of homocystine (HO)(=homocysteine-homocysteine) and homocysteine-cysteine disulphide (HO-CY), measured by Biotronik LC 2000 amino acid analyser, were compared with those in 20 obligate heterozygotes for HOA and in 40 controls matched for sex and menopausal status (1). The patients and the controls had normal renal and liver functions, and normal blood levels of vitamin B6 and folic acid.
Accepting HO and/or HO-CY peak levels after M-Loading exceeding the range of controls as indicating HOA, 18 out of the 20 obligate heterozygotes fulfilled this criterion. Surprisingly, 7 out of the 25 patients in the first group and 7 out of the 23 patients in the second group showed after-load peak levels of HO and/or HO-CY in the range of those in obligate heterozygotes. In none of the 14 patients in the third group excessive homocysteinemia was established. Final proof of heterozygosity for HOA as a risk factor of premature arteriosclerosis at young age, will depend on the measurements of enzyme activity in fibroblast cultures in these patients with excessive homocysteinemia after M-loading. In fact, cystathionine synthase activity was similar to that found in the obligate heterozygotes , in 4 of 5 cell lines studied so far from group i, and in 3 of 4 from group ii.

References:

1): G.H.J. Boers, e.a.: Unique efficiency of methionine metabolism in premenopausal women may protect against vascular disease in the reproductive years. J. Clin. Invest. 1984, in press.

## HYPERORNITHINEMIA WITH GYRATE ATROPHY OF THE CHOROID AND RETINA

*Harms, E., Gallasch, G.*

Universitäts-Kinderklinik und Universitäts-Augenklinik, 6900 Heidelberg, FRG

Three cases of hyperornithinemia with gyrate atrophy of the choroid and retina are presented. This autosomal-recessively inherited disorder is characterized by progressive deterioration of visual function first noted at school age and without treatment leading to total blindness during the fourth decade of life. Mental retardation is an inconstant finding in gyrate atrophy patients.
The metabolic defect of the disease is the lack of ornithine-$\delta$-aminotransferase which converts ornithine to glutamic acid and proline. In skin fibroblast cultures of our patients we found less than 5% activity for this enzyme compared to normal controls. No response to pyridoxine was noted either in vitro or in vivo . In one patient we could establish a low arginine diet by which plasma ornithine levels could be reduced to about half. Arginine is the only metabolic precursor of ornithine and an essential amino acid in patients with ornithine-$\delta$-aminotransferase deficiency. For the two and a half years of treatment until now, no further deterioration of visual function was noted. This finding supports other reports that reduction of plasma ornithine levels by a low arginine diet might be able to stop the fatal course of gyrate atrophy due to hyperornithinemia. Therefore, in retinopathy of unknown etiology in childhood a plasma amino acid analysis should be performed to detect hyperornithinemia at an early stage of the disease.

## RICHNER HANHART SYNDROME ALONG WITH MORBUS WILSON

*Overkamp*[1], D., *Jakober*[1], B., *Weidle*[2], E., *Thiel*[2], H.J., *Eggstein*[1], M.

Medizinische Universitätsklinik[1] and Universitäts-Augenklinik[2], D-7400 Tübingen, Schnarrenberg, West Germany

In the following case report one patient with two very rare inherited metabolic diseases is described. The first record of illness was in 1960 with running tears, redness of tarsal conjunctiva, thin crusts at the margin of eye lids and later on with central opaqueness of the cornea indicative of herpetiform dystrophy. In 1981 Kayser Fleischer rings and sunflower cataracts were detected on both eyes.

Peritoneoscopy followed by histological examination of liver biopsies showed a liver cirrhosis compatible with Morbus Wilson. We found decreased values of serum coeruloplasmin with 5 mg/dl and serum copper with 51 µg/dl, while the excretion of copper in urine was increased with 307 µg/24 hours. Serum tyrosine was increased excessively with 1200 µ mol/l and urine tyrosine with 1294 µ mol/24 hours, while the other amino acids were normal.

Using special clinical chemical tests it could be demonstrated, that Richner Hanhart Syndrome and Morbus Wilson seemed to be present without interdependence. We conclude, that these two very rare inborn errors of metabolism can be present simultaneously in one patient. The diagnoses are typically based upon ophthalmological symptoms and should be confirmed by clinical and clinical chemical examinations.

Special problems of differential diagnosis and treatment of the diseases are discussed.

## 2-METHYLACETOACETYL-CoA THIOLASE DEFICIENCY. IN VITRO STUDIES WITH DEUTERATED METABOLITES IN THREE PATIENTS

*Lehnert*, W., *Niederhoff*, H.

Universitäts-Kinderklinik, Mathildenstr.1, D-7800 Freiburg, FRG

2-methylacetoacetyl-CoA thiolase deficiency is a rare inborn error of isoleucine metabolism, associated with excretion of 2-methylacetoacetate, 3-hydroxy-2-

methylbutyrate and tiglylglycine. Diagnosis is made by detection of these metabolites by gas chromatography and gas chromatography-mass spectrometry. The patients present with lots of severe ketoacidoctic attacks following minor intercurrent infections or surgical interventions. By our selective screening for organic acidurias we diagnosed three cases with 2-methylacetoacetyl-CoA thiolase deficiency.
To study metabolic response to clinical condition and treatment in more detail, a method for quantification of the above mentioned metabolites was developed using deuterated internal standards and multiple ion detection gas chromatography-mass spectrometry. Synthesis of the deuterated compunds, the quantification procedure and results will be discussed.

## SENSITIVE, QUANTITATIVE, SIMPLE SCREENING TEST FOR ARGINASE DEFICIENCY

*Konarska L., Tomaszwewski, L.*

University Medical School, Department of Clinical Biochemistry, ul. Banacha 1, 02-097 Warsaw, Poland

Determination of arginase activity in erythrocytes is actually recommended as a main diagnostic parameter in an inherited arginase deficieny /hyperargininemia/. Arginase assay described here is based on measuremnt of ornithine produced by enzymatic hydrolysis of L-arginine. The blood /0.01 ml/ collected on filter paper is dried at room temperature. Thermostability of the enzyme enables to mail the specimens to a diagnostic center for testing. A disc /3 mm in diameter/ punched from dried blood specimen is deposited in a test tube where all further steps of estimation are performed: hemolysis and extraction from filter paper, activation of arginase with $Mn^{2+}$ at 55°C incubation with substrate at 37°C, and development of red colour with ninhydrin in a strong acid medium. The second disc of the same diameter is used for Hb determination. The activity is expressed in U/g Hb.
There was a good correlation /r = 0.954/ between activities determined in blood dried on filter paper and fresh erythrocytes of the same 150 blood specimens taken from normal adults. The activity was respectively 62.7 $\pm$ 15.7 and 62.5 $\pm$ 16.8. In 118 newborns the activity determined in dried blood spots was higher i.e. 101.9 $\pm$ 27.2.
In hyperargininemia, the activity of red cell arginase was found to be 0 - 10 %

of normal. Good precision, accuracy and sensivitiy make this method highly useful for screening purposes in newborns and older subjects.

## OXALATE DYNAMICS IN PRIMARY HYPEROXALURIA AND RENAL FAILURE

*Watts*[1], R.W.E., *Purkiss*[1], P., *Veall*[2], N.

[1]Divisions of Inherited Metabolic Diseases and [2]Radioisotopes, MRC Clinical Research Centre, Harrow, U.K.

Oxalate biosynthesis is increased in primary hyperoxaluria (PH) and the kidneys are destroyed by urolithiasis and nephrocalcinosis. Calcium oxalate is also deposited in other organs (oxalosis). Following a bolus injection of [$^{14}$C] oxalate and [$^{99m}$TC] diethylenediaminepentaacetate (DTPA), we measure the disappearance of $^{14}$C and $^{99m}$Tc from the blood and their appearance in the urine. The urinary oxalate ($U_{Ox}$) is also measured enzymatically. The following are calculated from the computer-simulated steady state plasma concentrations of the isotopes, their excretion into the urine over the whole period of the test and the urinary oxalate excretion: plasma oxalate concentration ($P_{Ox}$), oxalate distribution volume (ODV), oxalate metabolic pool size [(ODV) x ($P_{Ox}$)] , total plasma oxalate clearance ($PC_{Ox}$), renal (or dialyser or peritoneal) oxalate clearance ($RC_{Ox}$), non renal oxalate clearance ($NRC_{Ox}$) and the tissue oxalate accretion (TOA) rate. Negligible amounts of $^{14}$C are lost in the breath and faeces. Therefore, $NRC_{Ox}$ = [($PC_{Ox}$) - ($RC_{Ox}$)] and TOA = [($NCR_{Ox}$) x $P_{Ox}$)] . These derived values have been used to assess: (i) sequential changes in PH patients without overt renal failure; (ii) their size in PH patients requiring renal replacement; (iii) the contribution of the renal failure itself; (iv) the relative efficiencies of haemo- and peritioneal dialysis and of renal transplantation for the removal of oxalate.

Sequential values were unaltered over 3 years in 5 PH patients with no overt renal failure (GFR = 44-91 ml $min^{-1}$. 1.73 $m^{-2}$). TOA correlated with the clinical course in the individual patients. $RC_{Ox}$ and ODV were 2-3 times and about 1.5 times the GFR and ECF volume respectively in 5 normal subjects and in these patients. Haemodialysis removed oxalate more efficiently than peritoneal dialysis but neither could keep up with the TOA when performed for clinically acceptable times. Patients with PH and advanced renal failure have ODV and ECF values similar to those without overt renal failure and control subjects but $P_{Ox}$ and the oxalate metabolic pool are greatly increased. A case of PH studied 3 months after an apparently successful renal transplant showed that in spite of initial improvement $RC_{Ox}$ and GER were 7.7 and 5 ml $min^{-1}$. 1.73 $m^{-2}$ respectively although the other derived values still showed some improvement over the pretransplant results. The deterioration was associated with calcium oxalate nephrocalcinosis and not with immunological rejection. Hence, dialysis can only be of temporary help, and the prognosis with transplantation remains bad.

## A MITOCHONDIRAL MYOPATHY WITH A DEFICIENCY OF NADH-CoQ REDUCTASE ACTIVITY IN A MOTHER AND SON

*Busch, H.F.M., Scholte, H.R., Luyt-Houwen, I.E.M., Arts, W.F.M.*

Departments of Neurology, Biochemistry I and Pathology, Academic Hospital "Dijkzigt", Dr Molewaterplein 40, 3015 GD Rotterdam, The Netherland

Well-defined lesions of the respiratory chain may be found in some patients with myopathy and structural abnormalities of the muscle mitochondria. A deficiency of NADH-CoQ reductase activity may occur as a sporadic disorder, but it has been found in two sisters, which suggests a genetic origin[1].

A 42-y-old woman[2] experienced easy fatiguability and proximal weakness since the age of 32 y and her 15-y-old son had similar complaints since age 10 y. In both patients subsarcolemmal aggregates of abnormal mitochondria was the main structural abnormality in the muscle biopsy.

In muscle homogenates the activity of succinate dehydrogenase was 73% of control values in the mother and 215% in the son. Respective values for cytochrome c oxidase (measured with reduced cytochrome c) were 33% and 76%.

Mitochondrial fractions are isolated form freshly obtained biopsies. The respiratory rates with pyruvate, glutamate and palmitoylcarnitine (all plus malate) were reduced to 33%, 26% and 27% of average control rates in the mother and in the son to 14%, 11% and 18%. Succinate oxidation was resp. 63% and 84% of normal, while ascorbate oxidation was 44% and 50% of control rates. $Mg^{++}$-ATPase was normally stimulated by uncoupler. The activity of mitochondrial ß-oxidation measured as the conversion of [U-$^{14}$C] palmitate into $CO_2$ and perchloric acid soluble intermediates was normal.

The severe depression in the oxidation of the NAD-linked substrates appears to be main lesion and it proved to be more severe in the son. The decrease in as-

corbate oxidation is probably secondary. Interestingly, the total carnitine content of the muscle proved to be reduced in the mother to 36% of normal but it was 130% in the son, which suggests that the carnitine deficiency in the mother is secondary to the respiratory chain defect.
NADH-CoQ reductase deficiency may be genetically determined. In our family the molecular defect underlying this deficiency is likely to differ from that described by Morgan-Hughes[1], since we observed vertical transmission.

References:
1) J.A. Morgan-Hughes et al., 1979 J. neurol. Sci. 43; 27-46.
2) H.F.M. Busch et al., 1981 in: Mitochondria and muscular diseases. Eds. H.F.M. Busch, F.G.I. Jennekens and H.R. Scholte, Mefar B.V. Beetsterzwaag, The Netherlands, pp 207-211.

## A RIBOFLAVIN-RESPONSIVE PATIENT WITH GLUTARIC ACIDURIA TYPE II, AND HER THREE ASYMPTOMATIC SISTERS, ALL WITH A DEFECTIVE MITOCHONDRIAL BETA OXIDATION IN MUSCLE & FIBROBLASTS AND SEVERE SYSTEMIC CARNITINE DEFICIENCY

*Scholte[1], H.R., de Visser[2], M., Schutgens[3], R.B.H., Luyt-Houwen[1], I.E.M.*

Departments of Biochemistry I, Erasmus University (P.O. Box 1738, 3000 DR) Rotterdam; Neurology & Pediatrics, University of Amsterdam, The Netherlands

A 17-y-old girl suffering from a progressive, severe, overall reduction in muscle strength and muscle tonus, became bound to the wheel chair, and detoriated even further. Her respiratory muscles became barely sufficient.
After the finding of low muscle carnitine (0.40 µmol/g wet wt.), unsuccessful carnitine & prednisone therapy was instituted. The familiy members were investigated for plasma carnitine. In 3 sisters of 18, 13 and 7 y of age low free carnitine (13,9,6 µmol/l) and total carnitine (16,15,6 µmol/l, resp.) levels were found. In subsequent muscle biopsies of the sisters low total carnitine concentration was encountered (0.69, 0.28, 0.26 µmol/g wet wt., resp.). Moreover in the isolated muscle mitochondria a reduced beta oxidative activity was found, both measured as oxygen uptake with palmitoylcarnitine plus malate, and as the conversion of $|U-^{14}C|$ palmitate into $CO_2$ & perchloric acid soluble products.
In urine of the index patient a hyper-excretion of organic acids was found typical for glutaric aciduria type II.

These findings prompted to the institution of a therapy with riboflavin (3x10 mg/day), and a lower protein & fat and high carbohydrate diet. A rapid dramatic complete clinical improvement occurred.
Also in cultured fibroblasts suspensions a reduced mitochondrial beta oxidation was detected. In all sisters the reduction was of the same order of magnitude. We assume that all sisters have a systemic defect in electron transfer flavoprotein or its dehydrogenase, together needed for the transfer of reducing equivalents from all mitochondrial acyl-CoA dehydrogenases to coenzyme Q. The systemic carnitine deficieny is probably secondary to the sequestration of coenzyme A. The reduction in muscular carnitine is much more impressive than in another adult patient with glutaric aciduria type II (Dusheiko et al. New. Engl. J. Med. 301, 1979, 1405-9), and than in the juvenile form (Mooy et al. J. Inher. Metab. Dis., in press). An asymptomatic patient with severe carnitine deficiency has been detected in another familiy investigation in a collaborative study of our Departments. The symptomatic patient died. It is not likely that she suffered from glutaric aciduria type II (Scholte et al. J Neurol Sci 42, 1979, 87-101). Probably the precipitating factor of prolonged fasting did not occur in the asymptomatic patients.
Professor J. Bethlem and Professor H.F.M. Busch are acknowledged for their stimulating help and advice.
Het Princes Beatrix Fonds leverde financiele steun aan dit onderzoek in zowel Amsterdam als Rotterdam, en wordt hartelijk bedankt.

## **Short Communications,** Room C

WEDNESDAY, MARCH 7, 1984

GENETIC COUNSELLING
Chairman: J. D. Murken (München/FRG)

14.00 P. Clemens (Hamburg)
Newborn Screening for Phenylketonuria and Other Errors of Metabolism: Validation and Handling of Abnormal Results

14.15 L. D. Fairbanks, H. A. Simmonds, G. S. Morris, E. Carapella de Luca, R. J. Levinsky, C. H. Rodeck, R. L. K. Chapman (Roma/London)
Rapid Prenatal Diagnosis in Patients at Risk for Inherited Purine Disorders Associated with Immunodeficiency

14.30 F. Güttler, S. L. C. Woo (Glostrup/Houston)
Linkage of PKU- and HPA-Alleles with Human Phenylalanine Hydroxylase Locus Specific DNA-Polymorphisms

14.45 W. Höller, S. Scholz, D. Knorr, F. Bidlingmaier, E.-D. Albert (München)
Evidence for a Genetic Polymorphism in Congenital Adrenal Hyperplasia due to 21-Hydroxylase Deficiency and Identification of Two Allelic Variants Predicting Heterozygosity

15.00 W. D. Lehmann, P. Clemens, N. Theobald, H. C. Heinrich, R. Grüttner (Hamburg)
Detection of Heterozygous Carriers for Phenylketonuria Using a L-Phenylalanine Stable Isotope Loading Test

15.15 M. Owada, T. Sakiyama, O. Nishiya, T. Kitagawa (Tokyo)
Prenatal Diagnosis for Inborn Errors of Metabolism in Japan

15.30 R. B. H. Schutgens, H. v. d. Bosch, G. J. Romeyn, M. S. A. Heymans, R. J. A. Wanders (Amsterdam)
Prenatal Detection of Zellweger (Cerebro-Hepato-Renal) Syndrome

## NEWBORN SCREENING FOR PHENYLKETONURIA AND OTHER INBORN ERRORS OF METABOLISM: VALIDATION AND HANDLING OF ABNORMAL RESULTS

*Clemens, P.*

Department of Pediatrics, University of Hamburg, Martinistr. 52,
D-2000 Hamburg 20, F.R.G.

In Hamburg newborn-screening at the fifth day is done for phenylketonuria, galactosemia, maple sirup urine disease, homocystinuria and hypothyreoidism. We analysed all screening-tests of the last seven years. According to these results special criterias for validation of abnormal screening-test-findings are given. Depending on the special clinical data and on the grade of abnormality of the result in each case a special handling should be done.

## RAPID PRENATAL DIAGNOSIS IN PATIENTS AT RISK FOR INHERITED PURINE DISORDERS ASSOCIATED WITH IMMUNODEFICIENCY

*Fairbanks*, LD., Simmonds*, HA., Morris*, GS., Carapella de Luca**, E., Levinsky+, RJ., Rodeck++, Ch., Chapman°, RLK.*

* Purine Laboratory, Guy's Hospital, ** Institute Di Puericultura, University La Sapienza, Rome, Italy

+ Institute for Child Health, ++ Kings College Hospital

° Derby City Hospital

Adenosine deaminase (ADA) and purine nucleoside phosphorylase (PNP) are two enzymes which catalyse sequential steps in the degradation and recycling of purine nucleotides vital for many important processes in the body - chief of which are the processes of cell replication involving DNA, RNA and protein synthesis, as well as the provision of energy in the form of ATP which drives many essential cellular reactions.

Delection or either enzyme ist associated in the case of ADA with severe combined immunodeficiency (SCID) as distinct from PNP deficiency where predominantly T-cells are affected. To date no successful pharmacological or therapeutic regimes have been devised and affected children will die from overwhelming infection within the first few years of life unless a compatible bone-marrow transplant donor can be found.

In collaborative studies we have carried out prenatal diagnosis in four cases at risk for ADA deficiency, and the first ever prenatal diagnosis in PNP deficiency. Prenatal diagnosis has been carried out previously in ADA deficiency using amniotic fluids cells. We have developed sensitive techniques using foetal blood which have enabled us to determine whether the foetus was affected, by two separate means, within three hours. This ist not only more rapid than the time taken with amniotic cells (approximately two weeks) but in the two instances in ADA deficiency where we found the foetus was ADA deficient, the amniotic fluid cells failed to grow. We have also been investigating the application of these sensitive techniques using uncultured amniotic fluid cells and were able to make a diagnosis that a foetus at risk for PNP deficiency was not a homozygote for the defect. This war subsequently confirmed in cultured amniotic cells, and cord blood at the time of delivery of a healthy female infant.

## LINKAGE OF PKU- AND HPA-ALLELES WITH HUMAN PHENYLALANINE HYDROXYLASE LOCUS SPECIFIC DNA-POLYMORPHISMS

*Güttler, F., Savio L.C. Woo*

The John F. Kennedy Institute, DK-2600 Glostrup, Denmark, and Howard Hughes Medical Institute, Dept. of Cell Biology, Baylor College of Medicine, Houston, Texas, USA

Phenylalanine hydroxylase mRNA purified from rat liver was used for synthesis and cloning of ist cDNA. The rat liver cDNA probe was capable of hybridizing with human phenylalanine hydroxylase mRNA and used for screening of a human liver cDNA libery comprizing 100,000 independent transformants. Specific hybridization signals were obtained from four phenylalanine hydroxylase cDNA clones. Three of the inserted human cDNA fragments cover in combination the expressed sequences of the human-phenylalanine hydroxyglase gene. Genomic DNAs isolated from random Caucasians and digested by restriction enzymes yielded restriction fragment length polymorphisms (RFLP's) using a human phenylalanine hydroxylase cDNA probe.

Lymphocytes from 8 Danish families with benign hyperphenylalaninemia (HPA) and 27 Danish PKU-families with 1 or 2 affected children and unaffected siblings were analyzed by RFLP. The type of phenylalanine hydroxylase deficiency of the probands was insured by frequent recalculations of the phenylalanine intake. The combined phenotype of the parents based on phenylalanine loading tests was consistent with the phenylalanine tolerance of their affected child.
In all the families analysed it was possible to establish linkage of the restriction fragment pattern with the abnormal allele of the family. In families with two affected children the segregration of the abnormal allele and disease state was concordant. Allelic segregation between the proband and unaffected siblings were discordant in the families.
The powerful tool of haplotype analysis of the PKU-allele was documented. However, the haplotypes of all four phenylalanine hydroxylase genes in a particular family may not be identifiable by comparison with the proband alone. So, the probability at present of prenatal diagnosis and carrier detection may depend also on the availability of an unaffected sibling or grandparents. Genetic services will improve in the future with the identification of additional haplotypes.

## EVIDENCE FOR A GENETIC POLYMORPHISM IN CONGENITAL ADRENAL HYPERPLASIA DUE TO 21-HYDROXYLASE DEFICIENCY AND IDENTIFICATION OF TWO ALLELIC VARIANTS PREDICTING HETEROZYGOSITY

*Höller, W., Scholz, S., Knorr, D., Bidlingmaier, F., Albert, E.-D.*

Universitätskinderklinik München, Abteilung für Pädiatrische Endokrinologie
Lindwurmstr. 4, 8000 München 2, Federal Republic of Germany

ACTH-stimulation studies were performed on 244 relatives of patients with congenital adrenal hyperplasia (CAH) due to 21-hydroxylase deficiency.
Sixty of the latter represent salt-wasting (SW) cases, 61 the simple virilizing (SV) form, and 11 showed nonclassical late-onset (NC) symptoms. All family members also underwent human leukozyte antigen (HLA) typing. In spite of the fact that none of the relatives' group demonstrated clinical symptoms, biochemical evidence of CAH was found in 5 cases. Therefor they were designated as having cryptic CAH, a well described nonclassical variant of CAH. Moreover, the results suggest that there is at least one further type of this disease with only a very mild phenotypic expression. Although responses to ACTH-stimulation demon-

strate wide overlapping ranges, the mean values of the 17-hydroxyprogesterone increases are signifinantly higher (p .05) in genetically defined heterozygous relatives of SW-patients than in the respective members of SV- families. The results are consistent with those obtained from HLA-typing. The data confirm not only that there is a strong positive relationship between nonclassical CAH and HLA-B14, but they also indicate that the SW-state shows a nonrandom association to HLA-Bw47, whereas the SV-type is in linkage disequilibrium with B5(w51). Most of the subjects havong B14 carry the complete haplotype Aw33, B14, DR1, and most of those having Bw47 possess the total haplotype A3, Bw47, DR7. It is important to note that none of the proven normal haplotypes of the parents shows one of these determinants, so that they are supposed to represent always a disease state and to be of predictive value to the heterozygous state.

## DETECTION OF HETEROZYGOUS CARRIERS FOR PHENYLKETONURIA USING A L-PHENYLALANINE STABLE ISOTOPE LOADING TEST

*Lehmann, W.D., Clemens, P., Theobald, N., Heinrich, H.C., Grüttner, R.*

Dept. of Pediatrics and Physiological Chemistry, University of Hamburg, Martinistr. 52, D-2000 Hamburg 20, F.R.G.

For discrimination between normozygous subjects and carriers for phenylketonuria we used oral loading with 25 mg/kg of pentadeuterated L-phenylalanine. The test derives diverse types of data derived from plasma Phe and Tyr concentrations, especially ratios of total Phe/total Tyr and L-($^2H_5$)Phe/L-($^2H_4$)Tyr. These ratios both give minimal classification errors below 2 %.

## PRENATAL DIAGNOSIS FOR INBORN ERRORS OF METABOLISM IN JAPAN

*Misao Owada, Takeshi Sakiyama, Osamu Nishiya, Teruo Kitagawa*

Dept. of Pediatrics. Nihon University School of Medicine, 8, 1-chome, Kandasurugadai, Chiyoda-ku, Tokyo 101 Japan

During the past 15 years, noticeable progress has been made in the techniques of prenatal diagnosis in many countries including Japan. This paper presents the results of our experiences of prenatal diagnosis for inborn errors of metabolism compared with the findings of a nation-wide survey of prenatal diagnosis for inborn errors of metabolism.

Method: We have made 45 cases of prenatal diagnosis for various kinds of metabolic disorders during the period from 1972 until 1983. For most discrders prenatal diagnosis is currently accomplished by analysis of enzyme activities in cultured amniotic cells.

Nation-wide survey of prenatal diagnosis for metabolic disorders was done as follows. Primary inquiries were made at university hospitals as to whether or not any prenatal diagnosis for metabolic disorders had been performed. Then, 14 institutes having had experience in prenatal diagnosis, were given questionaries for all cases examined by July 1, 1981.

Results and Discussion: The results of our own experiences and the nation-wide survey is shown in the Table.

Table

| | Our Lab. | | Nation-wide survey | |
|---|---|---|---|---|
| Lipidoses | 31 | 68.9 % | 84 | 66.1 % |
| Mucopolysaccharidoses | 3 | 6.7 % | 12 | 9,4 % |
| Mucolipidoses | 9 | 20.0 % | 10 | 7.9 % |
| Others | 2 | 4.4 % | 21 | 16.5 % |
| Total | 45 | 100.0 % | 127 | 100.0 % |

The distribution of the disease in prenatal diagnosis are almost the same in our experience and the results of the nation-wide survey.

On the other hand, there are considerable differences in the distribution of the genetic metabolic disorders performed in prenatal diagnosis in Japan, the United States, and Western Europe. The cases prenatally examined for Gaucher disease and I-cell disease were relatively frequent in Japan, but Tay-Sachs disease, MPS and Krabbe were more frequent in Caucasians. This suggest that there may be a considerable difference in incidence of each metabolic disorders in Japanese and Caucasians. T. Kitagawa (Nihon Univ.), H. Yabuuchi, S. Tarui (Osaka Univ.), M. Arima (NCNMMD), Y. Eto (Jikei Univ.) K. Tada (Tohoku Univ.), T. Kusunoki (Kyoto Pre. Univ. Med.), Y. Suzuki (Tokyo Univ.) and T. Orii (Gifu Univ.) involved in the nation-wide survey.

## PRENATAL DETECTION OF ZELLWEBER (CEREBRO-HEPATO-RENAL) SYNDROME

*Schutgens, RBH., vd Bosch*, H., Romeyn, GJ., Heymans,HSA., Wanders, RJA.*

University Hospital Amsterdam. Dept. of Pediatrics and Laboratory of Biochemistry, University of Utrecht*

The Zellweger syndrome (ZS) is an autosomal recessive trait characterized clinically by a generalized hypotonia, a typical facial appearance, hepatomegaly, disturbances in liver function, renal cysts and severe psychomotor retardation. Biochemically the ZS ist characterized by disturbances in the metabolism of pipecolic acid, bile acids and very long chain fatty acids[1]. The disease is usually lethal with death occurring in the first year of life. Ultrastructural studies have demonstrated the absence of peroxisomes in the hepatocytes and renal proximal tubules of ZS patients. More recently, we found that plasmalogens (1-0-alk-1'-enyl-2-acylphosphoglycerides) are virtually absent in liver, kidney, brain, muscle and heart of Zellweger patients and lowered in erythocytes and fibroblasts[2]. As several key enzymes of plasmalogen biosynthesis in rodent liver an brain are known to be peroxisomal[3], we have tested the activity of one of these enzymes - dihydroxy-acetone phosphate acyltransferase (DHAP-AT) - in tissues of Zellweger Patients and controls. In liver homogenates of patients (n=4) the DHAP-AT activity ranged from 0.00 - 0.24 nmoles/h/mg protein, whereas in controls (n=6) the DHAP-AT activity was 1.26-3.44 nmoles/h/mg protein. In fibroblast homogenates of Zellweger patients (n=9) the DHAP-AT activity was $0.33 \pm 0.25$ nmoles/h/mg protein (mean$\pm$s.d.) (range 0.01-0.81) and in controls (n=27) 4.90+2.05 nmoles/h/mg protein (range 1.59-8.68). In cultured amniotic fluid cells of controls (n=12) DHAP-AT activity was $6.49 \pm 2.00$ nmoles/h/mg protein (range 3.86-8.73). The incorporation of [$1-{}^{14}C$]-hexadecanol in plasmalogens in intact fibroblasts from Zellweger patients was only 11 % of the total radioactivity incorporated in phospholipids of these cells against 45 % in controls. On the basis of these results we think that prenatal detection of Zellweger syndrome may be possible by measuring both DHAP-AT activity and [$1-{}^{14}C$]-hexadecanol incorporation into plasmalogens in cultured amniotic fluid cells.

References:

1. Moser HW et al J. Neurochem (1983)41: abstract 825C
2. Heymans HSA et al Eur J Pediatr (1983) in press
3. Hyjra AK and Bishop JE Ann NY Acad Sci (1982); 386: 170 - 181

## **Short Communications**, Room B

THURSDAY, MARCH 8, 1984

PHARMACOGENETICS
Chairman: H. Kampffmeyer (München/FRG)

9.00 H.W. Goedde, D.P. Agarwal (Hamburg)
Pharmacogenetic Basis of Alcohol Sensitivity

9.15 R. Dubbels, W. Schloot (Bremen)
Pharmacogenetic Aspects of Benoxinate Metabolism

9.30 A. M. Bardelli,G. Lasorella, L. Barberi, L. Biagini, M. Vanni (Siena)
Clioquinol and Optic Atrophy

INBORN ERRORS OF THE ADULT
Chairmen: H. Kampffmeyer, W. Gröbner (München/FRG)

9.45 P. Propping, W. Friedl, R. Winter, F. Reimer (Heidelberg/Weinsberg)
Screening for Three Mendalian Disorders among Adult Psychiatric Inpatients

10.00 K. MacDermot, J. Allsop, R. W. E. Watts (Harrow)
The Rate of Purine de novo Synthesis in Familial (Autosomal Dominant) Hyperuricaemic Nephropathy

10.15 S. Singh, I. Willers, K.R. Held, H.W. Goedde (Hamburg)
HPRT Variants: Correlation of Fibroblast HPRT Activity with Hypoxanthine Utilisation and Growth in Selection Media

10.30 Coffee Break

11.00 H.A. Simmonds, J.H. Stutchbury, D. R. Webster, R. W. Spencer, R.A. Fisher, M. Wooder, M.F.B. Grundy, B.M. Buckley (London/Truro/Birmingham)
Expression of Xanthinuria in Two Adult Females

11.15 N. Saha (Singapore)
Haematological Parameters in Relation to Haemoglobin and Glucose-6-Phosphate Dehydrogenase Phenotypes

11.30 Ch. Dwivedi, D. N. Singh, S. Hara (Nashville)
Acute Intermittant Porphyria

11.45 M. Doss, J. Schneider (Marburg)
Porphobilinogen Synthase ($\delta$-Aminolevulinic Acid Dehydratase) Defect in the Homozygous State as Cause of Acute Hepatic Porphyria

12.00 R. J. Desnick. L. Ustasiewicz, P. V. Tishler, P. Mustajoki (Boston/Helsinki)
Acute Intermittant Porphyria: Genetic Heterogenety ot the Porphobilinogen Deaminase Deficiency

12.15 A. C. Sewell, D. J. O'Sullivan, R. H. Evans, B. Calcraft (Newport)
Euthyroid Hyperthyroxinemia: A Case of Familial T4 Excess due to an Albumin Binding Variant

12.30 H. Sauer, A. Schalhorn, B. Wolf-Hornung, W. Wilmanns (München)
Metabolic Error of Folate Metabolism in an Adult Patient with Megaloblastic Anemia (Possibly Dihydrofolate-Reductase-Deficiency)

Lunch

# PHARMACOGENETIC BASIS OF ALCOHOL SENSITIVITY

*Goedde, H.W., Agarwal D.P.*

Institute of Human Genetics, University of Hamburg, Hamburg, F.R.G.

It is widely known that Orientals and American Indians of Mongoloid origin respond with severe alcohol intoxication (facial flush, vasodialation, increased heart rate, hot in stomach etc.) after drinking an acute dose of ethanol. Until now, the pharmacogenetic basis of this unusual drug response was not fully understood. Acetaldehyde is considered to be the main toxic compound responsible for pharmacological reactions to alcohol. In several investigations from different groups, flushing subjects were found to have higher blood acetaldehyde levels than non-flushing individuals.

Recently, we found that inherited deficiency of an isozyme of NAD-dependent aldehyde dehydrogenase (ALDH, E C 1.2.1.3) is responsible for the impaired aldehyde metabolism. This isozyme (ALDH I) has high affinity for acetaldehyde oxidation and its inherent absence leads to an accumulation of acetaldehyde which causes release of catecholamines leading to vasomotor symptoms. Our Population genetic data further show that this inborn error defect in alcohol metabolism is very prevalent among Asian Orientals and American Indians but was not found in Caucasians and Black races.

In our further investigations, we found that in Japan, a significantly low frequeny of isozyme deficiency was observed in alcoholic patients as compared to healthy controls. Thus, genetically determined aldehyde dehydrogenase polymorphism may be protective against alcohol abuse in individuals deficient in ALDH I isozyme by virtue of initial aversive reactions to alcohol intake. This work was supported by Stiftung Volkswagenwerk, Deutsche Forschungsgemeinschaft and Wilhelm-Sander Stiftung.

## PHARMACOGENETIC ASPECTS OF BENOXINATE METABOLISM

*Dubbels, R., Schloot, W.*

Centre of Human Genetics and Genetic Counselling, University of Bremen, NW 2, 2800 Bremen 33, FRG

The local anesthetic drug benoxinate is widely used in ophtalmology as topical anesthetic. Generally, benoxinate is tolerated well by patients, but a few side effects like conjunctivity and eczema of eyelids as well as serious ulcerations of the human cornea and loss of visual acuity have been abserved.
We have developed a simple and rapid spectrophotometric assay for testing hydrolysis of this drug and compared our data to benzoylcholinchloride hydrolysis by human pseudocholinesterase (PCHE). Using purified PCHE as well as plasma samples from healthy adult volunteers from different populations (Germans, Icelanders, Greeks, Indians, Hungarians and South African Blacks) positive correlations have been observed between the enzymatic hydrolysis values of both substrates.
On the other hand family studies failed to show a strict correlation between benoxinate and benzoylcholine hydrolysis in the presence of the inhibitors sodium fluoride and dibucaine which are used for PCHE phenotyping. This may indicate an altered benoxinate metabolism in this sample. Further metabolic studies revealed an acetylated product of benoxinate.
We suggest that benoxinate is metabolized by the enzymes PCHE or a very similar enzyme and furthermore by N-acetyltransferase, both display polymorphic activities in man.

## CLIOQUINOL AND OPTIC ATROPHY

*Bardelli, A.M., Lasorella, G., Barberi, L., Biagini, L., Vanni, M.*

Paediatric Ophthalmology Department, University of Siena-Italy

The ocular toxicity of Clioquinol and the association between this drug and myelo-optic neuropathy (SMON) is investigated in children.
The malabsorbtion syndrome's pathogenesis is also discussed alternatively.

# SCREENING FOR THREE MENDELIAN DISORDERS AMONG ADULT PSXCHIATRIC INPATIENTS

*Propping*[1], P., *Friedl*[1], W., *Winter*[2], R., *Reimer*[2], F.

[1]Institut für Humangenetik, University of Heidelberg, Neuenheimer Feld 328, D6900 Heidelberg, FRG

[2]Psychiatrisches Landeskrankenhaus, D 7102 Weinsberg, FRG

It is a general experience of medical genetics that common diseases (e.g. diabetes mellitus, atherosclerosis, mental retardation, convulsive disorders) frequently represent a disturbance in a final common pathway to which numerous mechanisms may contribute. In many psychiatric deseases, genetic factors are obviously involved. Since psychiatric nosology is mainly organized according to symptomatology, not etiology, it is very difficult to define genetic entities among psychiatric patients.

Some well-defined Mendelian disorders are known, however, that may present as psychiatric diseases in adults, at least for a number of years. Among these disorders, Wilson's disease (WD), acute intermittent porphyria (AIP), and the adult type of metachromatic leucodystropha (MLD) can be fairly reliably diagnosed by screening procedures.

In an ongoing study, all patients (age 18 - 60 years) who are consecutively admitted to a psychiatric state Hospital are routinely examined for the three diseases, irrespective of diagnosis.The determined parameters are: plasma ceruloplasmin (CP) level for WD, uroporphyrinogen-I-synthase (URO) activity in erythrocytes for AIP, arylsulfatase (ASA) activity in leucocytes for MLD. So far, 1200 patients were examined.

Results. In 6 patients, ASA values were compatible with MLD; in one Subject reexamined so far, the value was confirmed. - In 15 patients, URO values were suggestive of AIP; in two patients reexamined so far and the offspring of one subject the values were confirmed. - In 11 patients CP values were compatible with WD; in 7 patients so far reexamined, however, CP values were found normal. Additional measurements are required to exclude false positive values. If it can be successfully demonstrated that at least a small portion of psychiatric patients suffer from a defined genetic disease, this would not only be of conceptual importance but have therapeutic and preventive implications as well.

THE RATE OF PURINE DE NOVO SYNTHESIS IN FAMILIAL (AUTOSOMAL DOMINANT) HYPER-URICAEMIC NEPHROPATHY

*Mac Dermot, K., Allsop, J., Watts, R.W.E.*

Division of Inherited Metabolic Diseases, MRC Clinical Research Centre,Harrow, U.K.

We have studied five families in which hyperuricaemia, gout and renal failure occur together in early life with a familial pattern compatible with autosomal dominant inheritance. This suggests the possibility of a single enzyme defect expressing itself in the heterozygous state. Such a defect might produce the clinical phenotype by either accelerating purine de novo synthesis or reducing the net secretion of urate across the renal tubule epithelium. It is difficult to interpret the results of studies to determine if an alteration of renal tubule transport is the primary pathophysiological event when there is, or may be, renal damage. The patients usually present when there is already overtly impaired renal function. Two X-linked single enzyme defects which can produce this clinical phenotype are associated with accelerated purine de novo synthesis as judged by the time course of the incorporation of isotopically labelled precursor molecules into the urinary urate in vivo.
We have measured the rate of in vitro purine de novo synthesis in blood mononuclear cells (> 90% lymphocytes) from the affected members of the 5 families with autosomal dominant hyperuricaemic nephropathy and compared the results with those obtained in age and sex matched control subjects, patients with a matching degree of renal failure due to non immune complex renal disease and patients with a single enzyme defect [hypoxanthine phosphoribosyl transferase (EC 2.4.2.8) deficiency, Lesch-Nyhan syndrome] which is independently known to accelerate purine de novo synthesis on the basis of in vivo studies. The experimental method (the rate of [$^{14}$C] formate incorporation into the cell purines which were separated as silver complexes) was also validated by showing that it could assess the acceleration of purine de novo synthesis associated with phytohaemagglutinin induced lymphocyte transformation.

The rate of purine de novo synthesis was the same in the familial hyperuricaemic nephropathy patients, the normal controls and in the control patients with renal failure due to non immune complex renal disease, whereas, it was markedly accelerated in the Lesch-Nyhan syndrome patients. We conclude that purine de novo synthesis is not accelerated in familial hyperuricaemic nephropathy and suggest that the metabolic lesion is primarily a renal one which reduces the net tubular secretion of urate.

## HPRT VARIANTS: CORRELATION OF FIBROBLAST HPRT ACTIVITY WITH HYPOXANTHINE UTILISATION AND GROWTH IN SELECTION MEDIA

*Singh, S., Willers, I., Held, K.R., Goedde, H.W.*

Institute of Human Genetics, University of Hamburg, Butenfeld 32, 2000 Hamburg 54 (F.R.G.)

An attempt has been made to evaluate the results of the investigations of fibroblast cell lines from 19 patients with HPRT deficiency by studying various enzyme parameters and uptake of purine in conjunction with their growth pattern in various selection media. The results point to the presence of a further subtle heterogeneity among these cell lines. It can be concluded from this study that for a better biochemical characterisation of the various forms, along with the assay of the purine uptake and enzyme studies, a simultaneous determination of the proliferation pattern of the cells in the different selection media is quite necessary. This may have some implications towards the understanding of the vast heterogeneity observed in the clinical manifestation. This conclusion would be presented in detail on hand of one or two relevant case studies.

## EXPRESSION OF XANTHINURIA IN TWO ADULT FEMALES

*Simmonds*, HA., Stutchbury*, JH., Webster*, DR., Spencer+, RW., Fisher+, RA., Wooder+, M., Grundy+, MFB., Buckley@, BM.*

* Guy's Hospital, London, + Royal Cornwall Hospital, Truro, and
@Queen Elizabeth Hospital, Birmingham

Xanthinuria is a rare inherited disorder which has been identified generally in adults. Males have predominated over females and the majority of cases have been asymptomatic and identified only during routine screening. Stones have formed in 33%, with urolithiasis being a more common cause of presentation in young infants.

I.. this paper we report studies in two adult females who represent the extremes of presentation discussed above. One was a healthy woman first noted to be hypouricaemic during investigation of urinary tract infection in the third trimester of pregnancy. Investigation or urinary oxypurines confirmed that the patient was xanthinuric - xanthine was the principal purine base excreted and the urine also contained raised hypoxanthine levels (xanthine/hypoxanthine ratio 8.7:1). The curious factor was the finding of significant amounts of uric acid in the plasma and the excretion of 0.5 mmol uric acid per day in the urine. Such high levels of uric acid were contrary to our experience in other adult xanthinurics. For this reason we re-investigated this woman 6 weeks post partum - a time when plasma uric acid levels are reputedly at their highest in normal woman. Uric acid was now undetectable in plasma and had fallen to very low levels in urine. We believe the earlier results are indicative of the extent of foetal uric acid production, which is normally masked.

The second case was a 54 year old Lebanese woman who had a neprectomy for renal stones in 1964. In 1981 a smooth orange radio-opaque stone (mainly xanthine with a calcium oxalate core) was removed from the remaining kidney. The post-operative course was complicated and the patient went into terminal renal failure. this woman had spent most of her life in Mediterranean Countries where incidence of uric acid stones is much higher than in Northern Europe. Xanthine, like uric acid, is a very insoluble purine. The Clinical history in this case underlines the role of the environment in inherited disorders associated with the over-excretion of an insoluble end product. One would consequently expect more cases of the other inherited purine disorder associated with the excretion of an insoluble purine -2,8-dihydroxyadenine lithiasis - in this area. It is surprising that no such cases have as yet been reported from there.

## HAEMATOLOGICAL PARAMETERS IN RELATION TO HAEMOGLOBIN AND GLUCOSE-6-PHOSPHATE DEHYDROGENASE PHENOTYPES

*Saha, N.*

Department of Physiology, National University of Singapore, Singapore 0511

Five hundred and forty nine apparently healthy subjects (380 males and 169 females) of age 5-65 yrs were investigated to examine the influence of different haemoglobin and red cell glucose-6-phosphate dehydrogenase (G6PD) phenotypes on some haemotological parameters. Haemoglobin and G6PD phenotypes were determined by starch-gel electrophoresis and enzyme assays. Haemoglobin content (hb), packed cell volume (PCV), mean corpuscular haemoglobin concentration (MCHC), total white cell count (TLC), and erythrocyte sedimentation rate (ESR) were determined by standard electronic and other laboratory methods. The results showed that the haemotological parameters were not influenced by the presence of the sickle cell trait (n-42). However the subjects with raised level of $hbA_2$ (n-26) had a higher ($P= < 0.01$) level of hb ($13.8 \pm 0.39$ g/dl) and lower ($P < 0.005$) TLC ($5.67 \pm 0.37 \times 10^3/mm^3$) and ESR ($20.8 \pm 3.4$ mm/hr) compared with those having normal level of $hbA_2$ (hb - $12.5 \pm 0.12$; TLC - $7.01 \pm 2.20$ and ESR - $35.8 \pm 2.3$). The subjects with hbSS (12) had much lower levels of hb ($9.9 \pm 1.3$ g/dl, PCV ($32.2 \pm 4.1\%$), MCHC ($30.5 \pm 0.79\%$) and higher values of TLC ($10.2 \pm 5.7 \times 10^3/mm^3$) and ESR ($90.0 \pm 9.5$ mm/hr). Only male subjects with hbA phenotype were compared to examine the influence of G6PD alleles. G6PD deficient subjects ($Gd^{B-}$ and $Gd^{A-}$: n-30) had higher ($P < 0.005$) levels of hb ($14.7 \pm 0.34$ g/dl) and PCV ($46.1 \pm 1.0$ %) compared with those having normal enzyme activity ($Gd^{B+}$ and $Gd^{A+}$: hb - $13.0 \pm 0.16$ g/dl and PCV - $41.0 \pm 0,46$ %). There was no significant difference in haemotological values between $Gd^B$, $Gd^A$ and $Gd^{B(KHARTOUM)}$ alleles in either sex.

It may therefore be concluded that the presence of sickle cell trait, ß-thalassaemia trait or G6PD deficiency per se do not cause any haemotological deficiency; rather, they may have some selective advantage in the haemopoietic mechanism.

## ACUTE INTERMITTANT PORPHYRA

*Dwivedi, Ch., Singh, D.N., Hara, S.*

Department of Pediatrics, Meharry Medical College, Nashville, TN. 37208 USA

Acute Intermittant Porphyria is an autosomal dominant inborn error of metabolism associated with reduced hepatic uroporphyrinogen I synthetase activity which causes increased excretion of porphyrin precursor, delta amino levulinic acid and porphobilinogen. This report is to describe a family with Acute Intermittant Porphyria. The index patient (AO) was presented with frequent abdominal colic and psychosis. Delta amino levulinic acid and porphobilinogen were quantitated which were found to be 5490 and 3654 µg/24 hrs of urine respectively. Excretion of other porphyrins were within normal ranges. Uroporphyrinogen I synthetase was assayed which was 15 p moles uroporphyrin/mg protein/hr, approximatley 50 % of the activity of nonporphyrics. Similar studies were performed in available family members. Four members of family were identified with Acute Intermittant Porphyria. This data provide further evidence for a primary mutation affecting uroporphyrinogen I synthetase in Acute Intermittant Porphyria. Furthermore assay of red cell uroporphyrinogen I synthetase activity may be a reliable indicator of the heterozygous state. (Supported by Maternal and Child Health Care Grant #440 and NIH Grant # RR-08198).

## PORPHOBILINOGEN SYNTHASE (δ-AMINOLEVULINIC ACID DEHYDRATASE) DEFECT IN THE HOMOZYGOUS STATE AS CAUSE OF ACUTE HEPATIC PORPHYRIA

*Doss, M., Schneider, J.*

Clinical Biochemistry and Medical Policlinic of the Faculty of Medicine of the Philipp University, Deutschhausstraße 17 1/2, D-3550 Marburg, Federal Republic of Germany

In two male patients with acute hepatic porphyria and persisting paralysis, which increased in intensity intermittently, the activity of porphobilinogen synthase (PBG-S; δ-aminolevulinic acid dehydr(at)ase) was diminished in periphal erythrocytes and bone marrow cells below 3% of controls. In contrast, the activities of uroporphyrinogen synthase and decarboxylase were normal. Both patients have been excreting high quantities of δ-aminolevulinic acid and porphyrins, mainly coproporphyrin III, in urine for years. Lead intoxication and tyrosinemia could definitely be excluded. There was no experimental evidence for the existence of an inhibitor to PBG-S in urine, serum and erythrocytes from these two patients. Red cell PBG-S activity could not restored by addition both of dithiothreitol and zinc ions in contrast to lead intoxication.
The PBG-S deficiency was confirmed after DEAE cellulose chromatography: the concordance of relative and specific activity before and after chromatography of PBG-S from patients and controls differs from the findings in lead poisoning. A mutation of PBG-S probably at the level of the structural gene is concluded as the molecular basis of the inherited PBG-S defect porphyria. Since the relatives also show lower activities of PBG-S (~50% of controls), the disease of these two patients represents a new enzymatic type of inherited acute hepatic porphyria, the excretion profile of which is qualitatively completely different

from those of the known hereditary acute hepatic porphyrias. The PBG-S defect in the patients appears to be inherited as an autosomal recessive condition; patients with severe deficiency most likely are homozygous for the defective gene while the less severe deficiency reflects the heterozygous state.
Two families with asymptomatic PBG-S deficiency were studied.
The discovery of this new hereditary type of porphyria confirms the theory of overlapping Transition in the biochemical signs and clinical symptoms as well as analogies among the acute hepatic porphyrias and lead poisoning.

(The study was supported by the German Research Association.)

## ACUTE INTERMITTENT PORPHYRIA: GENETIC HETEROGENEITY OF THE PORPHOBILINOGEN DEAMINASE DEFICIENCY

*Desnick, R.J*., Ostasiewicz, L.*, Tishler, P.V.**, Mustajoki, P.[+]*

* Mount Sinai School of Medicine, New York, NY, USA, ** Harvard Medical School, Boston, MA, USA, and + University of Helsinki, Helsinki, Finnland

Previously, we demonstrated the occurrence of stable porphobilinogen deaminase (PBG-D) enzyme-substrate intermediates, A → E (J Biol Chem 255:1993,1980) and developed sensitive biochemical and immunologic methods for their resolution and quantitation (J Clin Invest 68:1, 1981). Using these techniques, we investigated the nature of the enzymatic defect in acute intermittent porphyria (AIP). The amount of cross-reacting immunologic material (CRIM) was determined in erythrocyte lysates from 109 AIP heterozygotes (hets) from 70 unrelated families (representing 17 different ethnic or demographic groups) by immunotitration and rocket immunoelectrophoresis with monospecific rabbit anti-human PBG-D IgG. When equal enzymatic activities were analyzed, no detectable differences in the amounts of CRIM were observed [CRIM/specific activity (SA)=1.0] in normal individuals or in 76 AIP hets from 59 families. In contrast, 33 AIP hets from 11 families had CRIM/SA rations of 1.6 or 5.2, indicating the presence of non-catalytic enzyme protein. The distributions of the A → E intermediates were determined by crossed-immunoelectrophoresis. In contrast to the characteristic pattern in normal and CRIM-negative lysates (A>B>C ≫ D>E), two different profiles were observed in the CRIM-positive kindreds. In 4 families (CRIM/SA=1.6) the profile of non-catalytic CRIM was B>A>C>D>E. In 7 other families (CRIM/SA=5.2), the profiles were C>B>D>E>A, presumably due to increased stability of the substrate-bound intermediates (B→E). These results are consistent with different allelic PBG-D gene mutations and provide evidence for molecular genetic heterogeneity in AIP.

## EUTHYROID HYPERTHYROXINEMIA:A CASE OF FAMILIAL T4 EXCESS DUE TO AN ALBUMIN BINDING VARIANT

*Sewell*[1], A.C., *O'Sullivan*[1], D.J., *Evans*[2], R.H., *Calcraft*[2], B.

Depts. of Biochemistry[1] and Medicine[2], Royal Gwent Hospital Newport, Gwent NPT 2UB, UK

Most cases of euthyroid hyperthyroxinemia are due to elevations of thyroxine binding globulin (TBG) either congenital, or due to the effects of oestrogens or drugs. Recently several families have been reported in which euthyroid hyperthyroxinemia is due to an inherited albumin variant. A 31 year old man presented with chest pain but no overt signs of thyroid disease. Free thyroxine (FT4) and total T4 (TT4) were consistently elevated with all other thyroid hormones within normal limits. A "T4 loading" test was performed at two concentrations of T4 using the patient's serum, the results of which were comparable to a known case of familial T4 excess. T4 binding studies using Scatchard analysis revealed an abnormal albumin binding constant. Family studies confirmed the findings in the proband's mother with probable autosomal dominant inheritance. The description of this rare, benign condition has aroused much discussion as to the validity of FT4 determinations using analogue methodology.

METABOLIC ERROR OF FOLATE METABOLISM IN AN ADULT PATIENT WITH MEGALOBLASTIC ANEMIA (POSSIBLY DIHYDROFOLATE-REDUCTASE-DEFICIENCY)

*Sauer, HJ., Schalhorn, A., Wolf-Hornung, B., Wilmanns, W.*

Medizinische Klinik III, Klinikum Großhadern, Ludwig-Maximilians-Universität München und Abteilung Klinische Hämatologie der Gesellschaft für Strahlen- und Umweltforschung mbH München

An anemia with macrocytosis in the peripheral blood and obvious megaloblastic bone marrow transformation was observed in a 28 years old woman. She was known to be anemic since their 6th year of life. Former treatments with vitamin B12 and folic acid were unsuccessful.

When thepatient was referred to our department, we found a normal vitamin B12 excretion test (Schilling-test), but an excessively high excretion of formimino-glutamic acid (Figlu-test) in the urine after an oral load with 10 gramms of histidine. While vitamin B12 and folic acid levels in the blood serum were normal, it was clear, that the patient had not a folic acid or vitamin B12 deficiency, but a disturbance of the folic acid metabolism. The bioavailability of metabolically active folic acid derivatives (tetrahydrofolic acid with activated one-carbon-units) was obviously reduced. This could be also demonstrated by in vitro tests with bone marrow cells: the incorporation of tritium labeled deoxyuridine (dUR) into the DNA was reduced and the incorporation of thymidine (dTR) was increased. So, the ratio of dUR/dTR-incorporation, which is an indicator for the disability to activate enough one-carbon-units, was reduced. This ratio could be corrected in vitro by supplementation of tetrahydrofolic acid derivatives, but not by the oxydized folic acid and not by vitamin B12. These results suggest a defect in the regeneration of tetrahydrofolic acidor their derivatives in vivo. A 50% reduction of the activity of the dihydrofolate-reductase in the cytosol of bone marrow cells is suspicious for the biochemical basis of this defect. Further investigations on this subject are ongoing.

Clinically, the patient got into a good remission with normalization of blood counts, bone marrow morphology and Figlu-excretion under the treatment with 5-formyl-tetrahydrofolic acid (Leucovorin). A rather high dose of 30 mg per day was necessary to maintain this remission.

## Short Communications, Room B

THURSDAY, MARCH 8, 1984

INBORN ERRORS OF THE ADULT
Chairman: P. Schwandt (München/FRG)

| | | |
|---|---|---|
| 14.15 | O. Sperling (Tel-Aviv)<br>Inborn Hypouricemia due to Isolated Defect in Renal Tubular Uric Acid Transport | |
| 14.30 | W. Mraz, H. Jatzkewitz (München)<br>The Activator(s) of Different Sphingolipid Hydrolases. Intracellular Distribution and Partial Characterization | |
| 14.45 | A. Lageron (Paris)<br>Adult Niemann-Pick Discase: Histoenzymological Data | |
| 15.00 | H.H. Goebel, I. Warlo (Mainz)<br>Ultrastructural Studies of the Skin in Neurometabolic Disorders | |
| 15.15 | H.A. Dresel, I. Otto, U. Frees, D.P. Via (Heidelberg/Houston)<br>Purification of Acetyl-LDL Receptor from Human Leucocytes an Weakly Acidid Protein of 190 000 D Molecular Weight | |
| 15.30 | C. Lemmen, G. Wolfram, N. Zöllner (München)<br>Familial Hypertriglyceridemia (FHT) and the Hormonal Regulation of Lipogenesis in Human Cell Cultures | |
| 15.45 | Coffee Break | |

16.15 E. Manzato, G. Baggio, G. Crepaldi (Padova)
The Plasma Lipoproteins in Familial Hyperchylomicronemia: Analysis by Zonal Ultracentrifugation

16.30 Ch. Keller, Th. Demant, S. Hailer, G. Wolfram, N. Zöllner (München)
Effects of Drugs and Plasma Exchange in a Patient with Homozygous Familial Hypercholesterolemia Confirmed by Tissue Culture

16.45 O. Adam, A. Wieczorek, G. Wolfram, N. Zöllner (München)
Lipoprotein-Dextran Interactions in Patients with Familial Hypercholesterolemia (FHC)

17.00 P. Weisweiler, V. Heinemann, P. Schwandt (München)
Changes in the Function of Apolipoprotein A-I in Hypertriglyceridemia

17.15 D. Bojanovski, R.E. Gregg, M.S. Meng, R. Ronan, L.A. Zech, J. Light, H.B. Brewer (Bethesda)
Metabolism of Human Pro-ApoA-I-Tangier (T) in Normal and Tangier Disease Subjects

17.30 E. Vergani, G.A. Giudici (Milan)
Bile Lipid Composition and Hemostatic Variables in Homozygous Analphalipoproteinemia (Tangier Disease)

## INBORN HYPOURICEMIA DUE TO ISOLATED DEFECT IN RENAL TUBULAR ACID TRANSPORT

*Sperling, O.*

Department of Clinical Biochemistry, Beilinson Medical Center, Petah-Tikva, and Department of Chemical Pathology, Tel-Hashomer, Tel-Aviv University Medical School, Israel

Inborn hypouricemia due to isolated renal tubular defect is a rare disorder. Since the first report in 1972, 10 families with this condition have been documented, of which 7 were from Israel. All the families from Israel were Sephardi Jews, 5 of them of Iraqi origin, one of Lybian origin and one of Turkish-Bulgarian origin. The mode of inheritance of this defect is autosomal recessive. Among the 10 families with this syndrome, 4 propositi had in addition hyperabsorptive hypercalciuria, and 4 had kidney stones composed of either uric acid or of calcium Salts. In one family the hypercalciuria was associated with decreased bone density. Mild hyperuricosuria appears to be common among the propositi with renal hypouricemia. The effects of probenecid and pyrazinamide on uric acid clearance in the patients suggest the existence of two types of renal tubular abnormalities underlying the syndrome: defective presecretory tubular urate reabsorption and defective total pre- and postsecretory tubular urate reabsorption.

## THE ACTIVATOR(S) OF DIFFERENT SPHINGOLIPID HYDROLASES. INTRACELLULAR DISTRIBUTION AND PARTIAL CHARACTERIZATION

*Mraz*, W., Jatzkewitz, H.,*

Max-Planck-Institut für Psychiatrie, Neurochemische Abteilung, München, Federal Republic of Germany

Various lysosomal sphingolipid hydrolases have been highly purified and characterized with synthetic substrate analogues. During purification these lysosomal enzymes lose their activity towards their physiological substrates. This activity can be restored in vitro by the addition of either ionic or non-ionic detergents or by (an) enzymatically inactive low molecular weight physiological activator protein(s). The results obtained during the study of the intracellular localization of the activator protein of cerebroside sulphatase (sulphatase A) can be summerized as follows:

1. An activator protein necessary for the enzymic hydrolysis cerebroside sulphate could be partially purified from unfractionated rat liver and proved to be a heat-stable, nondialyzable, low molecular weight protein with an isoelectric point of 4.1, the activity of which could be destroyed by pronase.

2. For elucidation of its subcellular distribution rat liver was fractionated by differential centrifugation. The intracellular distribution of the activator of cerebroside sulphatase was compared to the distribution patterns of marker enzymes for different cell organelles and found to coincide with the lysosomal arylsulphatase, thus indicating a lysosomal localization.

3. This was confirmed using highly purified, secondary, i.e., ironloaded, lysosomes. After disruption by osmotic shock, these organelles hydrolyzed cerebroside sulphate when incubations were performed under physiological conditions with endogenous, as well as exogenous sulphatase A as enzyme.

4. After subfractionation of the disrupted secondary lysosomes into membrane and lysosomal fractions by high speed centrifugation, it was found that the activator protein was exclusively associated with the lysosol, whereas the acid hydrolases were distributed differently between the two fractions.

5. The lysosol was further fractionated by semipreparative electrophoresis on polyacrilamide gels. Two protein fractions were obtained: a high molecular weight fraction, containing the activator-free acid hydrolases and a low molecular weight fraction, containing the enzyme-free activator of cerebroside sulphatase.

6. In addition to its effect on cerebroside sulphatase, this low molecular weight protein fraction also stimulated a number of other sphingolipid hydrolases, e.g., cerebroside galactosidase, cerebroside glucosidase, ß-N-acetylgalactosaminidase as well as sphingomyelinase (all associated with the high molecular weight fraction).

7. These observations clearly indicate that the enzymic degradation of sphingolipids in the lysosomes depends upon the presence of (a) low molecular weight activator protein(s), thus suggesting a special mechanism of sphingolipid hydrolysis within these organelles.

At present it cannot be decided whether a universal activator protein stimulates all the sphingolipid hydrolases, or if different molecular species with very similar properties activate the different hydrolytic reactions (or groups of sequential steps). Since the activator protein obtained seems to be heterogeneous, as revealed by its gel electophoretic behaviour, the latter possibility cannot be excluded.

The implications of our finding with respect to the pathogenesis of the different sphingolipidoses will be discussed.

*Present address: Institut für Klinische Chemie, Klinikum Großhadern, Universität München, Marchioninistraße 15, 8000 München 70, FRG.

## ADULT NIEMANN-PICK DISEASE: HISTOENZYMOLOGICAL DATA

*Lageron, A.*

INSERM, 184 rue duFg St-Antoine, 75012 Paris

Adult Niemann-Pick disease was diagnosed in our laboratory in 7 subjects aged from 15 to 27 years. The biopsy material studied was always the liver, and also, in 3 cases, bone marrow, spleen and kidney respectively. All tissues were analysed by histoenzymological techniques but sphingomyelinase was measured in leukocytes by a biochemical technique.

As regards the results for storage, the 7 patients formed 3 groups. The first group (3 cases) exhibited a typical B form in which phospholipids - mainly sphingomyelin - were intensively stored in macrophages, and hepatocytes participated in the storage (Baker and OTAN reactions with and without alkaline hydrolysis); a free cholesterol overload, only present in macrophages, was less abondant than the phospholipid overload (Schultz, oil red reactions). All 3 cases displayed greatly reduced sphigomyelinase activity but no neurological involvement. The second group (3 cases) also had decreased sphingomyelinase activity and no neurological injury, but only a little phospholipid storage in macrophages; hepatocytes were not overloaded by phospholipids and often contained less than the normal amount; but hepatocytes were intensively filled with free cholesterol also present in macrophages but to a lesser extent. This type of storage might constitute a special B form. In the last group (1 case) no storage occurred in hepatocytes but macrophages were greatly overloaded both by sphingomyelin and cholesterol. In this case, sphingomyelinase activity was normal but there was neurological involvement and vertical supranuclear ophtalmoplegia. This was therefore a C form of Niemann-Pick disease.

Despite these differences in storage, all 7 cases had common feature: - certain macrophages displayed monoaminooxidase and sorbitol dehydrogenase activity whereas other dehydrogenases were inactive, and hydrolase activity varied, - all viscera contained sea bleu histiocytes, - familial incidence was found: two cases were relatives uncle and nephew, and a brother of the C form patient had died of the same disease, - in the five cases where serum cholesterol was measured it was abnormally high. The last point underlines the close relationship between sphingomyelin and cholesterol metabolism in Niemann-Pick disease.

## ULTRASTRUCTURAL STUDIES OF THE SKIN IN NEUROMETABOLIC DISORDERS

*Goebel, H.H., Warlo, I.*

Division of Neuropathology, University of Mainz/FRG

While lymphocytes are a convenient population of cells for morphological, i.e. electronmicroscopic screening in lysosomal diseases shortcomings of their study comprise difficulty in preparing, i.e. isolating them and their limited involvement in metabolic conditions. Skin contains a multitude of different cell types, such as epidermal, eccrine and apocrine sweat gland epithelial, smooth muscle, and mural cells of dermal vessels as well as fibroblasts, Schwann cells and axons of dermal nerves, which provides a large spectrum of morphological lesions, properly identified only by electronmicroscopy, in such neurometabolic diseases as mucopolysacchatidoses, mucolipidoses, neuronal

ceroid lipofuscinoses, $GM_1$- and $GM_2$-gangliosidoses, metachromatic and Krabbe's leukodystophies, Niemann-Pick disease and neuroaxonal dystrophy.
This variation in dermal cytology permits high diagnostic morphological accuracy, both positive and negative, and renders biopsies of other tissues in neurometabolic disorders, but in very rare entities, rather unnecessary for morphological investigation.

## PURIFICATION OF ACETYL-LDL RECEPTOR FROM HUMAN LEUCOCYTES AN WEAKLY ACIDIC PROTEIN OF 190 000 D MOLECULAR WEIGHT

*Dresel*[1], HA., *Otto*[1], I., *Frees*[1], U., *Via* DP[2]

1: Medinzinische Klinik d. Universität Heidelberg
Bergheimerstraße 58 6900 Heidelberg FRG
2: Baylor College of Medicine, Dept. of Medicine
6565 Fannin A-601 Houston, Texas 77030 USA

We report a rapid three step scheme for purification of the acetyl-LDL receptor from human leukocytes (buffy coats). Preparation of Triton X-114 solubilized and detergent phase separated membrane proteins are subjected to ion exchanger chromatography (DEAE-, PEI-cellulose). Following elution from ion exchanger columne in Octylglucoside detergent is removed from receptor active fractions leaving the acetyl-LDL receptor in a soluble form. The receptor is than subjected to an affinity chromatography on acetyl-LDL coupled to Sepharose 4B. The receptor is eluted with PVS, a lately found inhibitor of acetyl-LDL-receptor interaction in the mouse system (Via, 1983). With this procedure a single acidic protein with a molecular weight of 190 000 D is isolated. The functional properties of the receptor will be discussed.

Via et al. (1983): New Aspects in Lipoprotein Metabolism
International Symposium of the Federation
of Cardiology Heidelberg 1983

## FAMILIAL HYPERTIGLYCERIDEMIA (FHT) AND THE HORMONAL REGULATION OF LIPOGENESIS IN HUMAN CELL CULTURES

*Lemmen, C., Wolfram, G., Zöllner, N.*

Medizinische Poliklinik der Universität München, 8 München 2,
Pettenkoferstr. 8a, BRD

The influence of insulin and triiodothyronine (T3) on lipogeneses was studied in different cell lines including fibroblasts from 8 patients with FHT. Addition of thyroid hormones to FHT cells caused a marked rise in acetate incorporation in triglyceride fatty acids, while there was no elevation in control cells. There was no change in cholesterol synthesis in adult normal and FHT cells under the same incubation conditions. Fibroblasts derived from fetal tissues (skin, lung) exhibited a similar rise in triglyceride synthesis following incubation with T3 as did the cells from patients with FHT. In contrast to FHT cells, cholesterol synthesis was also elevated in fetal fibroblasts following T3 treatment. With fibroblasts from human foreskin (newborn tissue) only a moderate T3 effect could be observed, whereas PHA stimulated lymphocytes from adult donors exhibited the "fetal pattern". Addition of insulin stimulated incorporation of acetate in triglyceride fatty acids in all cell lines mentioned above, with no significant difference between individual lines. There was no additive effect, when cells were incubated with insulin and T3 simultanously. Measurements of acetyl-CoA carboxylase activity in normal lines and in FHT cells supported the results obtained with acetate incorporation.

## THE PLASMA LIPOPROTEINS IN FAMILIAL HYPERCHYLOMICRONEMIA: ANALYSIS BY ZONAL ULTRACENTIFUGATION

*Manzato, E., Baggio, G., Crepaldi, G.*

Department of Internal Medicine - University of Padua -
Via Giustiniani, 2 - 35100 Padova - Italy

The object of this study was the analysis of plasma lipoproteins in 4 subjects with lipoprotein lipase deficiency and in two subjects with apo-C-II deficiency.

Lipoproteins were studied by zonal ultracentrifugation under rate flotation conditions and subclasses of VLDL, LDL, and HDL were isolated.

Lipoproteins of d $<$ 1.006 g/ml, and particularly lipoproteins with Sf $>$ 100, were present in very high concentrations. Low levels of d $>$ 1.006 g/ml lipoproteins were observed. This fraction was composed of some different and discrete lipoprotein populations: IDL (in 3 patients out of 6; d = 1.006-1.019 g/ml), $LDL_2$ (in all the patients; d = = 1.019-1.045 g/ml), $LDL_3$ (in all the patients; d = 1.045-1.063 g/ml), $HDL_2$ (in 4 patients out of 6), and $HDL_3$ (in all the patients).

$LDL_3$ were never observed in normal subjects by zonal ultracentrifugation; this LDL subclass seems to correspond to the LDL particles of very low Sf (2-5) previously identified in patients with type I and type V hyperlipoproteinemia by analytical ultracentrifugation. $LDL_3$ were isolated as a single and discrete peak in all the patients by means of zonal ultracentrifigation, thus allowing their physico-chemical characterization.

Lipoproteins of d $>$ 1.0006 g/ml were rich in triglycerides and poor in cholesterol in comparison with normal lipoproteins. The heterogeneity of LDL (particularly the appearance of $LDL_3$), the low levels of total HDL, and the lower $HDL_3$ flotation rate than the normal are typical aspects of serum lipoproteins in hypertriglyceridemic patients.

We did not find any significant difference in the lipoprotein profiles of the patients with lipoprotein lipase deficiency in comparison with apo-C-II deficiency. In both groups of patients, the plasma lipoprotein profile and the altered lipoprotein composition seems to be related to the impaired catabolism of triglyceride-rich lipoproteins due to the absence of lipoprotein lipase activity, while the presence of hepatic lipase activity could justify the abnormal properties of HDL.

EFFECTS OF DRUGS AND PLASMA EXCHANGE IN A PATIENT WITH HOMOZYGOUS FAMILIAL HYPERCHOLESTEROLEMIA CONFIRMED BY TISSUE CULTURE

*Keller, C., Demant, Th., Hailer, S., Wolfram, G., Zöllner, N.*

Medizinische Poliklinik der Universität München, Pettenkoferstr. 8a, D-8000 München 2, Germany

A 28 year old male was referred to us by the Dermatologic Department because of cutaneous xanthoma at both elbows in 1972. He had also tendinous xanthoma of the hands and the Achilles tendons were thickened. There were no definite symptoms of cardiovascular disease but arterial bruits over both femoral arteries could be heard. His serum cholesterol was 770 mg/dl. The family history for familial hypercholesterolemia (FHC) was negative except for one sister who had xanthomatosis of larger degree than the patient. Treatment with all lipid lowering drugs available was ineffective the serum cholesterol was never below 470 mg/dl. Later on tissue culture of skin fibroblasts confirmed receptor-defective homozygous FHC.

In 1974 a murmur of aortic insufficiency was noted and a systolic ejection murmur suggestive of left ventricular outflow tract obstruction. Occasionally ventricular extrasystoly was recorded in ECG. In 1979 ventricular arrhythmia became a therapeutical problem. By this time xanthoma had enlarged, new ones had developped and the corneal arcus lipoides was complete. Cardiac catheterization confirmed mild aortic insufficiency and a gradient of 20 mm Hg across the valve due to supravalvular narrowing. Diffuse coronary atherosclerosis was present and several stenoses up to 50 %.

Plasma exchange was started and has been carried out up to date. Nearly 60 treatments have been carried out uneventfully and approximately 550 g of cholesterol have been removed. Every fortnight plasmapheresis is done and 2.5 l of the patient's plasma are exchanged against a 5 % human albumin solution. The result is a rapid drainage of lipids and lipoproteins by 50 to 60 % compared to the concentration at the beginning of the procedure. Within two weeks the levels return to a value about 20 % below the initial concentrations before plasmapheresis was started. The addition of beta-pyridylcarbinol an alcohol corresponding to nicotinic acid with comparable effektiveness has not resulted in further decrease of lipids and lipoproteins nor in a decrease of rebound following plasma exchange. Clinical changes will be reported.

## LIPOPROTEIN - DEXTRAN INTERACTIONS IN PATIENTS WITH FAMILIAL HYPERCHOLESTEROLEMIA (FHC)

*Adam, O., Wieczorek, A., Wolfram, G., Zöllner, N.,*

Medizinische Poliklinik, Pettenkoferstr. 8a, 8000 München 2

By an infusion of dextrans (MW 40 000), used for hemodilution purposes, plasma cholesterol is lowered. In vitro interactions between dextrans and plasma lipoproteins have been demonstrated, yet little is known about factors contributing to the cholesterol-lowering effect of dextrans.

We investigated the effect of dextran-infusions in ten patients, admitted to our clinic, because of acute loss of hearing. They had been in good health before the event and gave their informed consent to the study.

Commercial available dextrans (MW 40 000) 500 ml/ d were infused over nine to twelve days. Cholesterol (Boehringer Mannheim, Germany) in plasma, VLDL, LDL and HDL, plasma volume (by labelling transferrin with indium) and routine laboratory tests (hematocrit, and plasma uric acid, protein and creatinine) were performed before and at the end of the treatment. Plasma volume was expanded by 300 ml and hematocrit and plasma protein decreased according to hemodilution. In comparison an exaggerated decrease of plasma cholesterol (-40 %) was found at the end of the treatment. Hypercholesterolemic patients revealed a greater decrease of plasma cholesterol, compared with normal controls.

This finding prompted an investigation into binding and internalisation of LDL to skin fibroblasts of normal controls and patients with FHC. The results of these studies revealed an enhanced binding and internalisation of dextran-treated LDL to skin fibroblasts, especially in patients with FHC.

In one patient, heterozygote for FHC, we monitored the timecourse of the dextran-effect on plasma cholesterol levels. After cessation of the dextran-infusion it took twelve days until plasma cholesterol regained preexperimental levels (345 mg/dl).

These data demonstrate a difference in cholesterol metabolism in patients suffering from FHC compared with normals, which becomes apparent under the conditions of dextran-infusions.

## CHANGES IN THE FUNCTION OF APOLIPOPROTEIN A-I IN HYPERTRIGLYCERIDEMIA

*Weisweiler, P., Heinemann, V., Schwandt, P.*

Medical Department II, Grosshadern Clinic, University of Munich,
Marchioninistraße 15, D-8000 Munich 70, FRG

Variants of the polymorphism of apolipoprotein A-I, the major protein constituent of high-density lipoproteins (HDL), may be one cause for an altered metabolism of serum lipoproteins. We studied apolipoprotein A-I isoforms in five normal subjects and in five patients with familial hypertriglyceridemia, by using fasting and postprandial serum samples.

Apolipoprotein A-I isoforms were characterized by the combination of SDS-electrophoresis and isoelectric focusing. The ability of apolipoprotein A-I to activate the enzyme lecithin: cholesterol acyltransferase (LCAT) was assayed by a purified enzyme preparation and liposomes.

In the postprandial state, the hypertriglyceridemic apolipoprotein A-I pattern was different from the normal pattern with an increase of the relative concentration of basic isoforms. The activity of the LCAT-enzyme could be less enhanced by hypertriglyceridemic apolipoprotein A-I than by normal apolipoprotein A-I.

Our results indicate that metabolic disturbances in hypertriglyceridemia may be partially due to changes in the function of apolipoprotein A-I.

## METABOLISM OF HUMAN ProapoA-$I_{Tangier\ (T)}$ IN NORMAL AND TANGIER DISEASE SUBJECTS

*Bojanovski, D., Gregg, R.e., Meng, M.S., Ronan, R., Zech., L.A., Light, J., Brewer Jr., H.B.,*

NIH, Bethesda, MD and WRAMC, Washington D.C., U.S.A.

Apolipoprotein (apo)A-I is the major protein moiety of human high density lipoproteins (HDL). Clinically, low plasma levels of apoA-I and HDL are associated with an increased risk of the development of premature cardiovascular disease. Several structural variants of apoA-I associated with low levels of plasma HDL have been recognized. Among them apo-A-I is of particular interest since it may provide insights into the biosynthesis and metabolism of human apo-A-I as well as HDL. Human apo-A-I is synthesized as a 267 amino acid preproapoA-I which initially undergoes intracellular co-translational proteolytic cleavage to proapoA-I. ProapoA-I, which contains a hexapeptide attached to the $NH_2$-terminous of mature apoA-I, is secreted into plasma. In normal subjects proapoA-I is rapidly converted to mature apoA-I in plasma by proteleytic cleavage. Normal human proapoA-$I_N$ us a relatively minor isoform in plasma. In Tangier diseass (TD) apoA-I is 5% of the normal plasma concentrations, but proapoA-I is a major plasma apoA-I isoform. This observation has led to the speculation that the abnormalitiy in TD is due to a defect in the conversion of proapoA-$I_T$ to mature apoA-$I_T$, and there is preferential rapid catabolism of the proapoA-$I_T$ leading to the low plama apoA-I level. In order to test this hypothesis, and further elucidate the defect in TD, the metabolism of proapoA-I isolated form normal and TD subjects were stuedied. ProapoA-I and proapoA-$I_T$ were radiolabeled with $^{131}I$ and $^{125}I$ respecitively and simultaneously injected into 2 normal and 1 TD subject. Radioactivity decay in plasma was determined and lipoproteins were isolated by ultracentrifuge (IEF) and the radioactivity in the isoforms quantitated. As determined by IEF the conversion of each propeptide in both normal subjects and TD patient to mature apoA-I was rapid and was completed within 12 hours. The comparison of their rates of catabolism form plasma revealed a significantly faster rate of catabolism of proapoA-$I_T$ than of proapoA-$I_N$ in both normal controls and TD patient. Similarly, the rate of catabolism of the mature apoA-$I_T$ was also faster than apoA-$I_N$ in both normal subjects and TD patient. The plasma residence times of proapoA-I were as follows:

| | ProapoA-$I_N$ | ProapoA-$I_T$ |
|---|---|---|
| Normal subjects (n=2) | 3.64 d | 1.03 d |
| Tangier patient (n=1) | 0.49 d | 0.37 d |

Plasma decay curves of simultaneously injected radiolabeled proapoA-I and mature apoA-I in normal or TD subjects revealed similar kinetic curves for the propeptide and mature isoforms, indicating very little, if any, preferential catabolism of the propeptide.

These results are consistent with the view that the defect in TD is not in the conversion of proapoA-$I_T$ to mature apoA-$I_T$ and that the rapid catabolism of both proapoA-$I_T$ and mature apoA-$I_T$ are responsible for the apoA-I and HDL deficiency in Tangier disease.

BILE LIPID COMPOSITION AND HEMOSTATIC VARIABLES IN HOMOZIGOUS ANALPHALIPOPROTEIN-EMIA (TANGIER DISEASE)

*Vergani, C., Giudici, G.A.*

Third Department of Clinical Medicine, University of Milan

We describe here a new case of HDL deficiency (Tangier disease). The proband had all the clinical, biochemical and histological hallmarks of the disease (yallow - orange tonsils, peripheral neuropathy, splenomegaly, low level of cholesterol, near absence of HDL-cholesterol and Apo A-I, accumulation of cholesteryl esters in the Schwan cell). The studies of the bile lipid composition in our patient showed that both hepatic and gallbladder bile were highly unsatured with cholesterol if compared with normal controls marked for sex, age and weight (2.4 % vs 6.6$\pm$1.5 % for hepatic bile, 3.5% vs 6.8 $\pm$ 1.4 % for gallbladder bile). In our patient the synthetic pathway of bile acids and the ratio between glyco and tauro conjugates were normal. Platelets studies showed that platelets underwent irreversible aggregation with low concentration of aggregating agents (ADP, collagen, arachidonic acid). The platelets produced higher amount of $TXB_2$ than control during aggregation induced by ADP, collagen thrombin and exogenous arachidonic acid. The relevance of these findings to the Glomset hypothesis of a reverse cholesterol transport in vivo from the periphery to the liver and to the clinical evidence of atherosclerotic lesions in pur proband will be discussed.

## **Short Communications,** Room C

THURSDAY, MARCH 8, 1984

MOLECULAR MECHANISMS
Chairman: W. Neupert, (München / FRG)

| | | |
|---|---|
| 9.00 | L. M. Steyn, E. H. Harley (Cape Town)<br>The Molecular Mechanism of Substrate Inhibition by Hypoxanthine of HPRT Cape Town |
| 9.15 | T. Ubuka, Y. Hosaki, R. Akagi, S. Kiguchi (Okayama)<br>Biosynthesis of 3-Mercaptolactate-Cysteine Disulfide |
| 9.30 | C. J. Danpure, P.R. Jennings, S. Halsall, T.J. Peters (Harrow)<br>Possible Vesicular Mechanism of Uptake an Intracellular Translocation of Cystine by Cystinotic Fibroblasts |
| 9.45 | A. J. C. Strydom,J. L. Meiring (Pretoria)<br>A Mechanism for the Tissue Damage in Homocystinuria |
| 10.00 | I. Kubota, M. Yoshino, S. Aramaki, C. Yasuoka, F. Yamashita, T. Saheki (Kogashima)<br>The Occurrence of a Mutant Arginase in Erythrocytes of a Patient with Argininemia |
| 10.15 | K. Tada, K. Hayasaka, Y. Igarashi (Sendai)<br>Molecular Lesion of Nonketotic Hyperglycinemia |
| 10.30 | Coffee Break |
| 11.00 | M. Hjellm, R. I. Kitney, J. Seakins (London)<br>Systems Analysis Applied to Metabolic Disorders. Methodological Aspects (I) |

11.15 J. W. Seakins, H. Hjelm, R. I. Kitney (London)
Systems Analysis of Phenylalanine Metabolism in Normal Subjects and Patients with Phenylketonuria (II)

11.30 J. D. S. Kay, D. Geiseler, V. Oberholzer, J. Seakins, M. Hjelm (London)
Systems Analysis of the Synthesis of Urea Following an Alanine Load in Normal Subjects and Patients with OTC Deficiency (III)

11.45 A. M. Vaccaro, M. Muscillo, K. Suzuki (New York)
Characterization of Glucosylsphingosine Glucosyl Hydrolase of Human Fibroblasts: Comparison with Glucosylgeramidase

12.00 J. Gehler, H. H. Goebel, M. Cantz, J. Spranger (Mainz / Heidelberg)
Clinical and Biochemical Findings in Neuraminic Acid Storage Disease (Salla Disease)

12.15 J. Baumkötter, K. Mendla, J. Gehler, J. Spranger, M. Cantz (Mainz)
Neuraminic Acid Storage Disease, Studies in Cultured Fibroblasts

Lunch

THE MOLECULAR MECHANISM OF SUBSTRATE INHIBITION BY HYPOXANTHINE OF HPRT

*Steyn, L.M., Harley, E.H.*

Department of Medical Microbiology and Department of Chemical Pathology, University of Cape Town Medical School, Observatory 7925, Cape Town, South Africa

Hypoxanthine-guanine phosphoribosyl transferase (HPRT) catalyses the transfer of ribose-5-phosphate from PP-ribose-P to the bases guanine and hypoxanthine to form their respective ribonucleotides, GMP and IMP, and pyrophosphate. The reaction mechanism is ordered random bi bi with PP-ribose-P binding before the purine base. We have described a variant form of HPRT in haemolysates from a patient with moderate purine overproduction. The predominant kinetic feature of this variant was substrate inhibition by guanine and hypoxanthine. The activity of the variant HPRT approached zero at high concentrations of the inhibitory substrates. This total inhibition suggested the formation of a dead-end complex between the enzyme and inhibitory substrate. When initial activity was measured at a number of fixed concentrations of the inhibitory substrate and the concentration of the non-inhibitory substrate, PP-ribose-P, was varied, a pattern of uncompetitive substrate inhibition was obtained on double reciprocal plots. This pattern can be expected when there is an ordered sequential addition of substrates,and supports the proposed mechanism for the normal enzyme. When assayed at high concentrations of the inhibitory substrate, in the presence of PPi at different fixed concentrations, a series of non-parallel lines, intersecting near the ordinate, was obtained. When assayed in the presence of IMP the enzyme activity gave a series of parallel lines. The interpretation of these patterns is that PPi and hypoxanthine interact on the enzyme to give enhanced inhibition, while hypoxanthine and IMP compete for the same form of the enzyme. From this data it is possible to postulate that the mechanism for substrate inhibition in this variant is the failure of PPi to dissociate from an abnormal E-base-PPi complex and the enzyme is trapped in this inactive form.

# BIOSYNTHESIS OF 3-MERCAPTOLACTATE-CYSTEINE DISULFIDE

*Toshihiko Ubuka, Yasuhiro Hosaki, Reiko Akagi, Shozo Kiguchi*

Department of Biochemistry, Okayama University Medical School, Okayama, 700, Japan

3-Mercaptolactate-cysteine disulfiduria is an inborn error of cysteine metabolism. Patients excrete large amounts of 3-mercaptolactate-cysteine disulfide (2-hydroxy-2-carboxyethylthio)cysteine) in the urine (Crawhall et al.,1968). Small amount of the disulfide is exreted in normal human urine (Ubuka et al., 1968). It has been reported that erythrocytes from these patients lack 3-mercaptopyruvate sulfurtransferase (Shih et al., 1977; Hannestad et al., 1981). As already reported, L-cysteine is metabolized, in part, via the transaminative pathway in rat tissues (Ubuka et al., 1977). The present study has been undertaken in order to elucidate the mechanism of the biosynthesis and the excretion of 3-mercaptolactate-cysteine disulfide.

The incubation of L-cysteine with $\alpha$-keto acid analog of L-cysteine, with rat heart homogenate also resulted in the formation of the disulfide. The formation of 3-mercaptolactate and cysteine from 3-mercaptopyruvate was detected at the same time. 3-Mercaptolactate-cysteine disulfide was formed when 3-mercaptolactate was incubated with rat heart homogenate. However, the disulfide was not formed when 3-mercaptopyruvate was incubated with liver or kidney homogenates, in which 3-mercaptopyruvate sulfurtransferase activity is very high. On the other hand, the activity of this enzyme was rather low in the rat heart. The disulfide was excreted in the urine of rats which were injected intraperitoneally with 3-mercaptolactate.

In conclusion, 3-mercaptolactate-cysteine disulfide seems to be formed by side reactions of the transaminative pathway of cysteine metabolis when 3-mercaptopyruvate sulfurtransferase activity is low, as in the rat heart, or is lacking as in these patients.

POSSIBLE VESICULAR MECHANISM OF UPTAKE AND INTRACELLULAR TRANSLOCATION OF CYSTINE BY CYSTINOTIC FIBROBLASTS

*Danpure, C.J., Jennings, P.R., Halsall, S., Peters, T.J.*

Divisions of Inherited Metabolic Diseases and Clinical Cell Biology, Clinical Research Centre, Watford Road, Harrow, Middlesex HAL 3UJ, UK

The lysosomal storage disease cystinosis is characterised by the intralysosomal accumulation of the amino acid cystine, due to an impaired cystine efflux from the lysosomes. Although much of the work on cultured cystinotic cells has involved the use of exogenously-added radioactive cystine, little is known about the mechanism by which extracellular cystine gains access to the intralysosomal compartment.

In an attempt to distinguish between 1) plasma membrane transport into the cystosol followed by transport across the lysosomal membrane into the lysosomes, and 2) endocytosis followed by fusion between the endosomes and lysosomes as two possible routes for cystine entry, confluent monolayers of normal and cystinotic human skin fibroblasts were cultured for varying periods of time from 3 min to 4 days in Hams F10 medium containing 15 % FCS and [$^{35}S$] cystine (12 - 36 µCi/ml, 130 µM). After harvesting and washing the cells, they were homogenised in 0.25 M sucrose containing 1 mM EDTA, pH 7.4. After spinning off the nuclei, the cytoplasmic fraction was layered onto a continuous sucrose gradient (SG 1.05 - 1.32) and spun at 4 ° for 35 min at 95,000 g. Fraktions were collected and analysed for marker enzymes and high and low molecular weight $^{35}S$. After adding NEM (10 mM) selected samples were subjected to automated amino acid analysis.

The results showed that even after very short labelling times (3 min) the majority (75%) of the radioactivity in cystinotic cells was in lysosomes or lysosome-like organelles. Practically all (93.6%) of the lysosomal label was in the form of cystine, while only 31.8% of the cystosolic label was cystine, the remainder being in the form of cysteine, glutathione and a variety of acidic metabolites.

The rapidity with which exogenous [$^{35}S$] cystine reaches a vesicular or lysosomal compartment in cystinotic cells is strongly indicative of an uptake route that bypasses the metabolic enzymes of the cytosol. The most obvious candidate for this is endocytosis followed by fusion of the endosomes with lysosomes. Failure of cystine efflux from the lysosomes in cystinotic cells would effectively limit the accessibility of the [$^{35}S$] to cystosolic metabolism. On the other hand cystosolic radioactivity probably results mainly from plasma membrane transport.

## A MECHANISM FOR THE TISSUE DAMAGE IN HOMOCYSTINURIA

*Strydom, A.J.C., Meiring, J.L.*

Department of Chemical Pathology, University of Pretoria, Box 2034, Pretoria, 00001, RSA

The basic pathology in homocystinuria is connective tissue damage. The object of the study was to develop a model which explains the damage.
Homocysteine has one methylene group more than cysteine in the side chain. It makes a remarkable difference to the pKa values and chemical reactivity of their respective -SH and $\alpha$-amino groups. At physiological pH, cysteine is oxidized at a faster rate than homocysteine. Disulphide exchange is much faster for homocysteine than for cysteine. Intra-molecular interactions of their respective reactive groups are responsible for the differences mentioned. Selective damage to structural proteins (especially connective tissue protein) by homocysteine under proper conditions is implied.
Recent findings proved the chemical composition of connective tissue in arteries, cartilage, brain, and eye to be similar in a high degree - specifically proteoglycans and link proteins. Binding action of these proteoglycans and link proteins depent on the integrity of their disulphide bonds. Disruption of links due to prolonged presence of homocysteine is the result.
Construction of a three dimensional molecular model explains the fibrous tissue damage even when homocysteine concentrations are relatively low.
This model may explain the start of atherosclerosis in people who are not genetically homocystinurics.

## THE OCCURRENCE OF A MUTANT ARGINASE IN ERYTHROCYTES OF A PATIENT WITH ARGININEMIA

*Kubota, K., Yoshino, M., Aramaki, S., Yasuoka, C., Yamashita, F., Saheki*, T.*

Department of Pediatrics, Kurume University, Kurume and
Department of Biochemistry, Kagoshima University*, Kagoshima, Japan

The deficiency of arginase activity has been demonstrated in erythrocytes of patients with argininemia. The mechanism of this enzyme deficiency has, however,

remained unknown. The present study was designed to elucidate the molecular basis of the enzyme deficiency in argininemia.
The arginase activity was determined by measuring urea splitted from arginine. For the immunochemical analyses, the antirat liver arginase antibody developed in the rabbitts was used. It was confirmed by the double immunodiffusion technique that this antibody cross reacts with purified human erythrocyte arginase as well as the rat liver enzyme.
The activity of arginase was not detected in the patient's hemolysate, and in the presumed heterozygotes, the activities ranged from 19 to 33% of the normal mean. The immunotitration studies revealed that the patient's hemolysate consumes the antibody and that the hemolysates from the presumed heterozygotes consume more amounts of the antibody per each unit of arginase activity than control. The Km values toward arginine, pH optima and the heat stability of the enzyme from the presumed heterozygotes did not differ significantly from those of normal control. The results of the immunotitration studies indicate that a catalitically inert, but antigenically active mutant arginase occurs in the hemolysate of the patient, and that normal arginase and the mutant enzyme probably coexist in the hemolysates of the heterozygotes. The enzymological characteristics of the heterozygotes' enzyme appear to represent almost exclusively those of normal enzyme.
These results are consistent with the autosomal recessive mode of inheritance of this trait.

## MOLECULAR LESION OF NONKETOTIC HYPERGLYCINEMIA

*Keiya Tada, Kiyoshi Hayasaka, Yutaka Igarashi*

Department of Pediatrics, Tohoku University Mediscal School - Sendai JAPAN

Nonketotic hyperglycinemia (NKH) is an inborn error of metabolism in which large amounts of glycine are found in body fluids. Most patients with NKH develop rapidly progressing neurological symtoms such as lethargy, muscular hypotonia, respiratory distress or convulsions in neonatal period and die within few weeks, whereas the survivors are handicapped with severe psychomotor retardation.
In 1969, we demonstrated that glycine cleavage system (GCS) was defective in the livers from the patients with nonketotic hyperglycinemia. GCS is composed of four protein components: P-protein which is a pyridoxal phosphate-dpendent glycine decarboxylase, H-protein which is a lipoic acid containing protein, T-protein which is a tetrahydrofolate-requiring protein, and L-protein which is a

lipoamide dehydrogenase. Therefore, the disturbance in GCS could be by a defect in any of these four components. However, which component is particulary defective in nonketotic hyperglycinemia has been obscure.
Recently we had the opportunitiy to investigate the individual component of GCS in the liver and brain obtained from two autopsied cases of nonketotic hyperglycinemia.
The overall activity of GCS was found to be extremely low in both the liver and brain of each patient. In one patient, only the activity of P-protein was undetectable both in the liver and brain. Immunochemical analysis indicated that this resulted from an absence of the enzyme protein. In the other patient, only the activity of the T-protein was undetectable in the liver and brain. These findings suggest that nonketotic hyperglycinemia may result form defect in any one of the enzyme components of GCS and that an individual component protein of GCS is controlled by the same gene both in the liver and brain.

## SYSTEMS ANALYSIS APPLIED TO METABOLIC DISORDERS. METHODOLOGICAL ASPECTS (I)

*Hjelm*[1], M., *Kitney*[2], R.I., *Seakins*[1], J.

Institute of Child Health[1] and Imperial College[2], University of London, UK

Systems analysis is ancient as a concept but has only recently been introduced as a tool in dealing with complex biological situations such as the regulation of blood pressure (1), carbohydrate metabolism (2) the synthesis of acute-phase proteins (3) and recently metabolic disorders (4). This development has been greatly facilitated by the rapid progress in computer technology involving simulations studies of even very complex situations. The principal steps in systems analysis of intermediary metabolism are to: -

1. define the purpose of the analysis, e.g. to elucidate the relationship between plasma concentrations of metabolites in terms of their turnover at organ level or to estimate metabolite concentrations in tissues not accessible to direct measurements.

2. establish an appropriate biochemical and physiological model based on present available knowledge and reasonable assumptions.

3. translate the conceptual model into a computer model which comprises the mathematical equations describing the functional relationships.

4. validate the computer model from a structural point of view, e.g. that concentrations are positive, that the total amounts in a closed system stay constant, and that the results of computer simulation are in agreement with available biological data.

5. design trials for biological validation of the model using computer simulation.

6. perform biological validation and to compare predicted and experimental results.

7. refine the model based on the outcome of the previous steps.

Systems analysis promotes a powerful integration between theoretical work and trials and can considerably increase the interpretation of clinical data in functional terms.
The metabolism of phenylalanine in normal subjects and in patients with PKU, and the synthesis of urea following an alanine load are two clinical examples which illustrate the advantages and disadvantages of this approach.

1) Kitney, R.I. J. Biomed Eng. 1979, Vol. 1, No 2, 89-99
2) Finkelstein, L. and Carson, E. R. Mathematical Modelling of Dynamic Biological Systems. 1979.
3) Groth, T. Hyltoft Petersen P, and Hjelm M. Comp. Prog. Biomed. 1978, 8, 295-300.
4) Hjelm, M., Kitney, R.K., Lindsey, P. and Seakins, J. Submitted for publication.

SYSTEMS ANALYSIS OF PHENYLALANINE METABOLISM IN NORMAL SUBJECTS AND PATIENTS WITH PHENYLKETONURIA (II)

*Seakins*[1], J.W., *Hjelm*[1], M., *Kitney*[2], R.I.

Institute of Child Health[1] and Imperial College[2], University of London UK

The techniques of systems analysis and computer simulation habe been applied to a wide variety of metabolic problems, but apart from a study of the urea cycle have not been applied to inborn errors of metabolism (1).
We describe the application of these techniques to phenylalanine metabolism. The model consists of four biological functions, digestion and absorption, protein synthesis and breakdown, catabolism and elimination of phenylalanine and its metabolites and interorgan transport, and contains seven lumped compartments, liver, kidney, muscle, brain (target organ), intestines, metabolically inactive space and plasma (mixing). Enzyme reactions are assumed to obey Michaelis-Menten kinetics; and the effects of transport delays, and diffusion through the blood brain are ingnored, although the model is designed to incorporate the appropriate functions as required.

The computer model has potential for estimating concentrations of key metabolites in human organs which are not accessible to direct analysis from measurements of metabolites in blood and urine and phenylalanine intake. Such estimates could be helpful in clinical decisions concerning modification or termination of dietary treatment. The model could also be used to obtain realistic in vivo values for enzyme rate constants etc. and to devise investigations to determine the quantitative importance of the auxiliary pathways in phenylalanine metabolism in PKU.

The model has been successfully validated using data from single and continuous intravenous loads on normal subjects (2) from PKU patients on normal diets (3) and from a patient during relaxation of the diet (4).

1) C. Bachman and J. P. Columbo. Enzyme 1981, <u>26</u>, 259-264
2) S. Rödger. MD Thesis, Göteborg, 1977
3) S. K. Wadman, C. Van der Heiden, D. Ketting and F.J. Van Sprang. Chlin. Chim. Acta, 1971, <u>34</u>, 277-284
4) J. W. Seakins, R. S. Ersser and M. Jhelm. J. Inher. Metab. Dis. 1982, <u>5</u> Supp. 19-20

SYSTEMS ANALYSIS OF THE SYNTHESIS OF UREA FOLLOWING AN ALANINE LOAD IN NORMAL SUBJECTS AND PATIENTS WITH OTC DEFICIENCY (III)

*Kay, J.D.S., Geiseler, D., Oberholzer, V., Seakins, J., Hjelm, M.*

Institute of Child Health, University of London, U.K.

Previous approaches to measuring of the rate of urea synthesis in man have depended on timed urine collections or the use of isotopes. If a suitable dose of alanine is given to a human the rate of synthesis of urea and its concentration in plasma increases. Systems analysis of this situation indicated that a single compartment model could be assumed, as (a) most cell membranes are freely permeable to urea, and (b) there is no catabolic pathway for the compound. With this formulation the synthesis rate of urea is proportional to the change of its concentration within the lumped compartment and can be derived from timed measurements of the plasma concentration of urea. Two parameters can be derived in order to characterise urea synthesis after an alanine load, $\hat{f}$ = the maximum synthesis rate, and $\hat{t}$ = the time of the maximum synthesis rate.

Computer simulation was used in predicting the errors in the synthesis parameters introduced by such factors as frequency of specimen collection, varying distribution volume and urinary excretion rate and analytical imprecision.

A simple practical procedure could be worked out based on these results and used for the biological validation of the model. This was carried out by establishing the dose-response curve for urea synthesis after oral and intravenous alanine in healthy subjects and the kinetics of urea synthesis in female obligate heterozygotes for ornithine transcarbamylase deficiency. In the first group values for $\hat{f}$ were in close agreement with those reported in the literature. Results in obligate heterozygotes indicate two biochemically different situations, a decreased $\hat{f}$ at a normal $\hat{t}$ and a normal $\hat{f}$ at an increased $\hat{t}$.

CHARACTERIZATION OF GLUCOSYLSPHINGOSINE GLUCOSYL HYDROLASE OF HUMAN FIBROBLASTS: COMPARISON WITH GLUCOSYLCERAMIDASE

*Vaccaro, A.M., Muscillo, M., Suzuki, K.*

Laboratory of Metabolism and Pathological Biochemistry, Instituto Superiore di Sanita, 00161 Rome, Italy, and Departments of Neurology and Neuroscience, and the R. F. Kennedy Center, Albert Einstein College of Medicine, Bronx, N.Y. 10461, U.S.A.

Gaucher disease is an autosomal recessive disorder due to a deficiency of glucosylceramidase activity. Accumulation of glucosylceramide occurs in tissues of patients. Recently, presence of glucosylsphingosine (glucopsychosine), which is not found in normal tissues, has been reported in the spleen and brain of some patients. Absence of glucosylsphingosine glucosyl hydrolase has also been abserved in the spleen and fibroblasts of Gaucher patients. The nature of the enzymatic hydrolysis of gluco-psychosine has not been studied in detail, nor has it been completely established that glucosylceramide and glucosylsphingosine are hydrolyzed by the same enzyme. We have studied the properties of the glucosylsphingosine glucosyl hydrolase of human fibroblasts and have compared them with those of glucosyl-ceramidase. The standard assay systems to measure the two enzymatic activities contained sodium taurocholate (0.25% w/v) and oleic acid (0.025% w/v). The two activities showed many differences. The pH optima were 4.8 for psychosine hydrolysis and 5.3 for glucosylceramide hydrolysis. In the presence of oleic acid, taurocholate activated glucosylceramidase more than 10-fold, while it activated psychosine hydrolysis only by about 30%. When taurocholate was substituted by crude brain phospatidylinositol, glucosyl-ceramidase activity decreased by 50%, while psychosine hydrolysis increased by 20%. Triton X-100 was stimulatory for glucosylceramidase but was strongly inhibitory for psychosine hydrolysis. The Km values for the two substrates were similar; $1.7\mathrm{x}10^{-5}$M for psychosine and $3.0\mathrm{x}10^{-5}$M for glucosylceramide. The Vmax for glucosylceramide was however 80 times that for psychosine hydrolysis. Psychosine acted as a potent non-competitive inhibitor (ki = $1.1\mathrm{x}10^{-5}$M), while glucosylceramide was a weak inhibitor against glucosylsphingosine hydrolysis. Within the limit of glucosyl ceramide solubility, psychosine hydrolysis could not be inhibited by more than 50%. Furthermore, the Dixon plot of glucosylceramidase inhibition showed an anomalous slope. These findings cast some doubt on the hypothesis that both of these substrates are hydrolyzed by a single enzyme through the same catalytic or binding site. Since hydrolysis of both substrates ist blocked in Gaucher tissues, it seems most likely that they are hydrolyzed by a single enzyme with two binding and possibly two catalytic sites for the respective substrates.

## CLINICAL AND BIOCHEMICAL FINDINGS IN NEURAMINIC ACID STORAGE DISEASE (SALLA DISEASE).

*Gehler*[1], J., *Goebel*[2], H.H., *Cantz*[3], M., *Spranger*[1], J.

[1]Kinderklinik und Abteilung für Neuropathologie der Universität, D-6500 Mainz,FRG.
[3]Institut für Pathochemie und Allgemeine Neurochemie der Universität, D-6900 Heidelberg, FRG

Salla disease is a lysosomal storage disease with a disturbed sialic acid catabolism. Until now, the underlying enzyme defect is not known. About 40 patients with this disorder have been published, all of them from Northern Finland. The main clinical symptoms are mental retardation, dwarfism and neurologic symptoms.

We report on a 3 5/12 year old boy of Italian descent, who developed clinical and biochemical symptoms of Salla disease. He is the 3rd child of consaguineous parents from Sicily, his birth weight was 4800 gm, birth length 52 cm. Immediately after birth, hepatosplenomegaly was noticed, and there were respiratory problems. At 10 months of age facial dysmorphism, marked motor retardation, hypotonia became obvious. At 20 months the boy showed a somewhat thickened skin with puffy eyelids and severe psychomotor retardation. Radiologically there were abnormal vertebrae and poorly modeled metacarpals. Peripheral blood smear showed vacuolated lymphocytes.
Electron microscopy of a skin biopsy revealed numerous cells with membrane-bound enlarged vacuoles, which containded finegranular material. Lysosomal enzymes and $^{45}SO_4$ incorporation in skin fibroblasts were normal.
The patient's urine showed a 25-fold increase of free sialic acid. Sialic acid was elevated in fibroblasts and leucocytes as well.
To our knowledge, our patient is the first case with Salla disease outside Finland. In contrast to the Finnish esperience, early hepatosplenomegaly and osteodysplasia were found in our patient.

NEURAMINIC ACID STORAGE DISEASE. STUDIES IN CULTURED FIBROBLASTS

*Baumkötter*[1], J., *Mendla*[1], K., *Gehler*[2], J., *Spranger*[2], J., *Cantz*[1], M.

[1]Institut für Pathochemie und Allgemeine Neurochemie der Universität,
D-6900 Heidelberg, FRG
[2]Kinderklinik der Universität, D-6500 Mainz, FRG

Fibroblasts cultured from a 2-year-old Italian boy with a neurodegenerative disorder were found to contain about 16 times the normal amount of free (unbound) sialic acid, identified by thin-layer chromatography as N-acetylneuraminic acid. Incubation of the cultures in the presence of the glycoprotein fetuin, tritium-labelled in its sialic acid portion, led to an efficient uptake. In the patients' fibroblasts, there was an abnormal accumulation of trichloroacetic acid (TCA)-soluble radioactivity, wheras the TCA-precipitable radioactivity was the same as in control cells. In chase experiments, the rate of disappearance of the TCA-soluble radioactive material was very much decreased as compared to the control cells. Upon gel chromatography, the major portion of the TCA-soluble radioactive material was eluted in a position identical to N-acetylneuraminic acid.

The results suggest that the lysosomal catabolism of the sialoglycoprotein is normal , but that the cellular release of the liberated sialic acid is somehow impaired, perhaps due to a defective lysosomal transport mechanism, a possibility first suggested by Renlund et al. (Eur. J. Biochem. 130, 39-45 (1983).

## **Short Communications,** Room C

THURSDAY, MARCH 8, 1984

NUTRITION AND GENETIC DISEASE
Chairman: W. Endres (München/FRG)

14.00 W. Blom, G.B. van den Berg, J. G. M. Huijmans, J. A. R. Sanders-Woudstra (Rotterdam)
Successful Nicotinamide Treatment in an Autosomal Dominant Behavioral and Psychiatric Disorder

14.15 M. Fràter-Schröder, P. Krieg, L. Kierat, J. Erten (Zürich)
Unexpected Secretion of a Transcobalamin II-like Vitamin B 12-Binding Serum Protein in Amniotic Fluid Cell Cultures

14.30 A. M. Bardelli, G. Lasorella, L. Barberi, L. Biagini, A.E. Speri (Siena)

Beta Carotene and Retinol in Mesodermal Ocular Pathology

14.45 A. M. Bardelli, L. Barberi, G. Lasorella, A. Fois (Siena)
Tyrosinaemia and Eye

15.00 F. K. Trefz, H. Schmidt, G. Pecht, M. Mahle, H. Bickel (Heidelberg)
Oral Loading Studies with Deuterated Phenylalanine in Heterozygotes of Phenylketonuria/Hyperphenylalaninemia

## Late Comers' Session I

Chairman: W. Endres (München/FRG)

15.15 R. Steinherz, N. Makov, R. Narinski, B. Meidan, G. Kohn (Peta-Tikva, Rehovot, Jerusalem)
Comparative Study of Cystine Accumulation and Clearance in Cystinotic and I-Cell Fibroblasts Upon Exposure to Cystine Dimethyl Ester.

15.30 L. Konarska, L. Tomaszewski, J.P. Colombo, H.G. Terheggen (Warsau, Bern, Köln)
Saliva - New Convenient Material for Detection of Hyperargininemia.

15.45 Coffee Break

16.15 A. Niederwieser, N. Blau, P. Joller, M. Atarés, J. Cardesa-Garcia (Zürich, Badjoz)
A New Variant of Tetrahydrobiopterin-Deficient Hyperphenylalaninemia: GTP Cyclohydrolase I Deficiency

16.30 E. Solem, C. Pirzer, O. Romero-Saravia (Frankfurt)
Mass Screening for Glusoce-6-Phosphate Dehydrogenase Deficiency: Clinical Implications. The Detection of New Isoenzymes.

SUCCESSFUL NICOTINAMIDE TREATMENT IN AN AUTOSOMAL DOMINANT BEHAVIORAL AND PSYCHIATRIC DISORDER

*Blom, W., van den Berg, G.B., Huijmans, J.G.M., Sanders-Woudstra*, J.A.R.*

Department of pediatrics (metabolic laboratory) and *childpsychiatry, Academic Hospital Rotterdam, Sophia Children's Hospital, Gordelweg 160, 3038 GE Rotterdam, The Netherlands

We discovered a family with an autosomal dominant behavioral an psychiatric disorder:

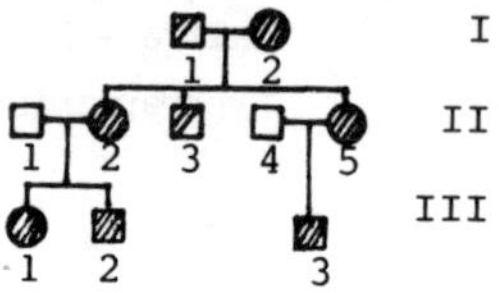

- I 1: Hot-tempered, alcohol abuse.
- I 2: As child difficult. Uncommunicative, contact disability, hot-tempered, atopic eczema.
- II 2: As child fits of crying and temper. Now restless, overactive and over-talkative. Sometimes dizziness.
- II 3: As child difficult. Now intermittendly depressive an fits of temper.
- II 5: As child fits of crying and temper. Later labile, stress sensitive. Was admitted to a psychiatric institute.
- III 1,2,3: In general:
  Unmanagable behavior, contact and play disability, hyperactive, restless, chaotic, agressive, stress-sensitive, fits of crying and temper.
  In addition:
  - III 1: Under-temperature during the first months of life. Extreme sleep difficulties. Atopic eczema (self-destructive scratching). At 5 years of age she wanted to be dead.
  - III 2: Ataxia and intention tremor.
  - III 3: Extreme sleep difficulties. Wanted to be a girl.

The children III 1,2 and 3 showed metabolically a picture of tryptophan malabsorption with increased urinary indican. On a tryptophan loading-test they had a tryptophan-metabolite pattern in urine suggesting a partial block in the kynurenine-pathway at the level of kynureninase.
On nicotinamide therapy they improved dramatically and in a couple of months they were clinically as good as normalized. They now receive 20 mg of nicotinamide/kg in 6 doses. At lower doses the clinical problems return.
Metabolic investigation in urine was done by TLC, HPLC and GCMS. A pedegree has been made for the five last generations. All the results will be shown and discussed.

UNEXPECTED SECRETION OF A TRANSCOBALAMIN II-LIKE VITAMIN B12-BINDING SERUM IN AMNIOTIC FLUID CELL CULTURES

*Frater-Schröder, M., Krieg, P., Kierat, L., Erten, J.*

Dept. of Pediatrics, University of Zürich, CH 8032 Zürich, Switzerland

Children with congenital transcobalamin II(TC2) deficiency are healthy at birth and develop severe hematological and immunological symptoms shortly after birth, that can be fatal if the patients are left on a normal unsupplemented diet. This suggests that TC2 cannot be an essential factor before birth. Contrary to expectations it was recently found that cordblood TC2 is of foetal origin and that the foetus may be capable of TC2 synthesis at least at the end of pregnancy (Blood 62: 234, 1983). It has been shown that human cultured skin fibroblasts synthesize and secrete TC2 (Schweiz. med. Wschr. 112: 1435, 1982). The question arose if foetal cells can synthesize TC2 as well.

Eight individual cell cultures derived from amniotic fluid were investigated using 1) solid-phase immunoassay (RIA) to detect total immunoreactive TC2 and 2) gelfiltration (G-150) after labeling with radioactive vitamin B12 (cobalamin) in order to separate the different B12-Binding proteins, in the concentrated cell culture medium.

At cell confluency (passage 2 or 3) amniotic cells secreted substantial amounts of immunoreactive TC2, that could be quantitated as apo TC2 by gelfiltration as well. In all eight cases a TC2-like fraction was detected. Phenotyping of the TC2-like fractions is in progress and will help to characterize the TC2-like molecule more precisely. A comparison with maternal TC2 serumtypes will then be possible.

The finding of TC2-like activity in prenatal cell cultures implicates a corresponding role for foetal TC2 in cobalamin utilisation of the foetus at earlier stages of development as well, and appears to contradict that fact that normal foetal development occurs in spite of the congenital absence of TC2. Thus the question as to how foetal cobalamin transport is regulated, remains unanswered.

## BETA CAROTENE AND RETINOL IN MESODERMAL OCULAR PATHOLOGY

*Bardelli, A.M., Lasorella, G., Barberi, L., Biagini, L., Speri, A.E.*

Paediatric Opthalmology Department. University of Siena -Italy-

Low levels of betacarotene and retinol are found in aniridia, congenital glaucoma and other mesodermal ocular pathology. The correlation between ocular and laboratory findings is discussed.

## TYROSINAEMIA AND EYE

*Bardelli, A.M., Barberi, L., Lasorella, G., Fois, A.,*

Paediatric Ophthalmology Department. University of Siena -Italy

Some cases of tyrosinaemia with eye and skin lesions are described. The diagnosis of type tyrosinaemia was based upon an increase of blood tyrosine, tyrosinuria and absence of liver and kidney abnormalities. The treatment with a low tyrosine phenilalanine diet has resulted in a disappearance of the ocular and systemic manifestations.

## ORAL LOADING STUDIES WITH DEUTERATED PHENYLALANINE IN HETEROZYGOTES OF PHENYLKETONURIA/HYPERPHENYLALANINEMIA

*Trefz, F.K., Schmidt, H., Pecht, G., Mahle, M., Bickel, H.*

Univ. Childrens Hospital, Im Neuenheimer Feld 150, D-6900 Heidelberg, GFR

Up to now there exist only few data concerning the biochemical state of heterozygotes of phenylketonuria (PKU) and of hyperphenylalaninemia (HPA). There is also an increasing interest in an accurate standardised test for detecting heterozygocity. In 15 heterozygotes of PKU / HPA oral loading tests with L-$d_5$-phenylalanine (30 mg/kg BW) were performed. The increase of deuterated phenylalanine and tyrosine in plasma was measured by gaschromatography/ massfragmentography. Molar ratios of phe / tyr were calculated 30 - 240 minutes after load. Best discrimination of the phe / tyr ratios compared to controls assumed to be homozygous for the wild type gene was found 30 and 120 minutes after load (table):

| | 30 | 240 minutes after load |
|---|---|---|
| Controls n = 7 | 5 - 9 | 3 - 5 |
| Heterozygotes n = 15 | 11 - 55 | 6 - 12 |

Table: Molar ratios of $d_5$-phenylalanine/$d_4$-tyrosine (range) in plasma 30 and 240 minutes after loading with $d_5$-phenylalanine

This method of genotyping was applied in three couples at risk for heterozygocity of PKW. Though this approach seems promising, more data are necessary to establish firmly the advantage of this test.

## COMPARATIVE STUDY OF CYSTINE ACCUMULATION AND CLEARANCE IN CYSTINOTIC AND I-CELL FIBROBLASTS UPON EXPOSURE TO CYSTINE DIMETHYL ESTER

*Steinherz*[1,2], R., *Makov*[2], N., *Narinski*[1], R., *Meidan*[3], B., *Kohn*[3], G.

Department of Pediatrics A, Beilinson Medical Centre, Petah-Tikva, Israel;
Department of Organic Chemistry, Weizmann Institute of Science Rehovot, Israel;
Department of Human Genetics, Hebrew University Medical School, Jerusalem,Israel

I-cell fibroblasts accumulate cystine at levels comparable to those seen in homozygous cystinotic fibroblasts. To examine whether the same mechanism, or two different unrelated defects, cause this phenomenon, we exposed cystinotic and I-cell fibroblasts to radioactive cystine dimethyl ester and looked at the rate of clearance of the accumulated radioactive cystine. Using this technique a defect in cystine clearance from cystinotic lysosomes in situ was observed (Proc. Natl. Acad. Sci. 79:4446-50, 1982). Comparison of cysteine-N-ethylmaleimide (=NEM) to cystine ratio and cysteine-NEM to cystine mono or dimethyl ester ratios between cystinotic and I-cell fibroblasts showed normal cysteine production in I-cell fibroblasts. Presumably, by cyctoplasmic reduction of the cystine generated within the lysosome by esterases. Although cystine clearance was found to be normal, accumulation of cystine mono and dimethyl esters observed in I-cell fibroblasts indicating reduction in esterase activity. The alkyl ester accumulation subsides getting longer period into clearance. We conclude that two unrelated mechanisms lead to cystine accumulation in I-cell and cystinotic fibroblasts and there is no defect in cystine clearance in situ in I-cell fibroblasts.

## SALIVA - NEW CONVENIENT MATERIAL FOR DETECTION OF HYPERARGININEMIA

*Konarska, L., Tomaszewski, L., Colombo*, J.P., Terheggen**, H.G.*

Medical School, Dept. of Clin.Biochemistry, ul. Banacha 1, 02-097 Warsaw, Poland, *Dept. of Clin.Chemistry, Inselspital Bern, Switzerland, ** Children's Hospital, Cologne, W.Germany

Arginase from normal human mixed saliva was characterized and a simple method for its determination was developed. The enzyme required preincubation with $Mn^{2+}$ at a final concentration of 5 mmol/l, for 20 min, at 55°C for complete activation. The pH optimum was 9.6 - 9.8. $K_m$ for L-arginine as a substrate was 4.2 ± 0,7 mmol/l. In normal saliva only one form of arginase was found. It was chromatographically identical with the cationic form of arginase demonstrated in liver and blood cells. Salivary arginase was completely precipitated by rabbit antiserum against purified human liver arginase.

We demonstrated arginase deficiency in saliva of patients suffering from hyperargininemia. The residual arginase activity in saliva of 3 hyperargininemia homozygotes was 0,4%/I.W./, 0,6% / A.W./, and 6% /M.W./ of normal subjects activity. Activity in saliva of heterozygous mother, father and healthy daughter was 0.082, 0.066 and 0.121 unit/mg protein, whereas the activity in saliva of 60 healthy adults and 8 children was 0.168 ± 0.113 and 0.161 ± 0.058 unit/mg protein, respectively.

Kinetic, chromatographic and immunological similarities of liver, blood cells and saliva arginases suggested their genetic identity. Deficiency of arginase in saliva, blood cells and liver in hyperargininemia provides a clinical evidence that these proteins could be specified by the same locus.

# A NEW VARIANT OF TETRAHYDROBIOPTERIN-DEFICIENT HYPERPHENYLALANINEMIA: GTP CYCLOHYDROLASE I DEFICIENCY

Niederwieser*, A., Blau*, N., Joller*, P., Atarés*, M., Cardesa-Garcia*, J.

*Department of Pediatrics, University of Zurich, Zurich, Switzerland.
**Hospital of Mother and Child, and Faculty of Medicine, University of Extremadura, Badajoz, Spain

A 4-year old patient with hyperphenylalaninemia, severe retardation in development, severe hypotonia, convulsions, and frequent episodes of hyperthermia without infections excreted abnormally low amounts of biopterin, neopterin, dopamine and serotonin in the urine and responded to oral loading tests with tetrahydrobiopterin by normalization of the elevated serum phenylalanine concentration.
Measurement of enzyme activities in liver biopsies have shown that the girl is sufferin from GTP cyclohydrolase I deficiency (activity was less than 4% of the mean of 10 controls). Enzyme activities in phytohemagglutinine-stimulated lymphocytes from patient, father and mother were zero, 32, an 49%, respectively, of the mean of four controls. GTP cyclohydrolase I converts GTP into dihydroneopterin triphosphate and formic acid, the first step in biosynthesis of tetrahydrobiopterin.
It was concluded that our patient is the first case of a new variant of tetrahydrobiopterin-deficient hyperphenylalaninemia and that this enzyme defect is inherited autosomal recessively. The metabolic defect ist an interesting model with respect to speculations that pterins, like neopterin, might actively participate in immunological processes.

MASS SCREENING FOR GLUCOSE-6-PHOSPHATE DEHYDROGENASE DEFICIENCY: CLINICAL IMPLICATIONS. THE DETECTION OF NEW ISOENZYMES

*Solem, E., Pirzer, C., Romero-Saravia, O.*

Zentrum der Kinderheilkunde, Universitätskliniken Frankfurt am Main, Theodor-Stern-Kai 7, D-6000 Frankfurt am Main 70

Glucose-6-Phosphate dehydrogenase (G-6-PD) deficiency is the most frequent desease-inducing enzyme defect in man. Depending on the type of G-6-PD-variant (ca. 150 different variants are known) the deficient persons develope prolonged neonatal jaundice, favism and medicament induced hemolytic anemia to a certain percentage, partly known in mediterranean countries. Mass screnning for G-6-PD deficiency was until now connected with problems. An improved screening method made it possible to eliminate false positive results,and detects more than 50 % of female heterozygotes. In Hessen 60.000 newborns were screened with the improved Beutler-flourescenz-spot-test and precise quantitative examinations, detecting more than 95 % of all heterozygote gene carriers were carried out in family examinations. A frequency of deficient neweborns of 1:250 was found. This finding correlates well with the high number of foreigners from the mediterranean area living in Hessen. Thus, this enzyme defect is more common than expected in this part of Middle-Europe.

Ca. 12 % of the deficient persons (including family members) were found to have, or had previously had hemolytic anemia. Several patients with hemolytic crisis, making transfusion treatment necessary were observed. Family examinations included the investigation of several parameters indicating hemolysis, showing that a light anemia was frequent in female heterozygotes.

Isoelectric focusing of red blood cell G-6-PD was investigated, giving at least 15 new bands of isoenzymes. The focused pattern of G-6-PD isoenzymes gives evidence of a multiallelic coding for this enzyme and opens new possibilities for typing G-6-PD-variants.

## **Short Communications,** Room B

FRIDAY, MARCH 9, 1984

NUTRITION AND GENETIC DISEASE
Chairman: B. Hadorn (München/FRG)

| | |
|---|---|
| 9.00 | W. Endres, R. Schaller, Th. Noss, R. Wörnle, Y.S.Shin (München)<br>Lethal Metabolic Disorders of the Urea Cycle. Argininemia and Argininosuccinic Aciduria. Sensitive Methods for Arginase and Argininosuccinic Lyase Assays using 14C-Arginine |
| 9.15 | A. Otten, U. Bürger, C. Bachmann, U. Hillig, H. Wolf (Giessen/Bern)<br>Late Diagnosis of and Therapeutical Approach to the Hyper-ammonemia-Hyperornithinemia-Homocitrillinuria Syndrome |
| 9.30 | J.-L. Dhondt, J.-P. Farriaux (Lille)<br>Relationship between Dietary Phenylalanine Tolerance and Biochemical Parameters of the Estimation of Phenylalanine Hydroxylase Activity |
| 9.45 | D. J. Byrd, H. Heinbokel, S. Schweitzer, J. Brodehl (Hannover)<br>Evaluation of Oral L-Cysteine for Treatment of Cystine Deficiency in Homocystinuria |
| 10.00 | R. Longhi, E. Riva, A. Rottoli, S. Paccanelli, C. Buttè, R. Valsasina, M. Giovannini (Milano)<br>Nutritional Control in PKU Children on Restricted Diet. The Trace Elements |
| 10.15 | I. Matsuda, A. Kitano, A. Higashi, N. Nagata, Y. Hase (Osaka)<br>Zinc Status of Histidinemic Patients |

10.30 Coffee Break

11.00 R. Infante, I. Beucler, M. E. Bouma, J. Schmitz, N. Amit (Paris)
Anderson's Disease. An Inborn Error of Intestinal Lipid Transport

11.15 A. C. Beynen, M. B. Katan, L. F. M. van Zutphen (Wageningen / Utrecht)
Differences in Individual Responce of Serum Cholesterol to Dietary Cholesterol in Rats, Rabbits and Man

11.30 S.-Di Donato, D. Pelucchetti, M. Rimoldi (Milano)
Systemic Carnitine Deficiency (SDC) in Two Adult Sisters: Full Reccovery with L-Carnitine Supplementation

11.45 H. S. Füeßl, F.-D. Goebel (München)
Clinical Variability of Maturity-Onset Type Diabetes of Young People (MODY)

12.00 Y. S. Shin, K. Ullrich, H. Kopp, M. Rieth, A. von Rücker, W. Endres (München / Münster)
Diagnosis of Various Types of Glycogen Storage Diseases with Blood Samples. Increased Amylo-1,6- -Glucosidase Activity in Erythrocytes in Glycogenosis VIa

12,15 S. Berlow, G. Hoganson, S. Kaufman, J. Muenzer (Madison/ Bethesda)
Treatment of Defects in Biopterin Metabolism

# LETHAL METABOLIC DISORDERS OF THE UREA CYCLE. ARGININEMIA AND ARGININOSUCCINIC ACIDURIA. SENSITIVE METHODS FOR ARGINASE AND ARGININOSUCCINIC LYASE ASSAYS USING $^{14}$C-ARGININE

*Endres, W., Schaller, R., Noss*[+]*, Th., Wörnle*[+]*, R., Shin, Y.S.*

Kinderklinik and Kinderpoliklinik[+], Univ. of Munich, F. R. G.

A 6 month-old male infant with severe cerebral palsy and growth retardation was found to have hyperargininemia and hyperammonemia (patient 1). A 5 day-old baby girl with severe convulsions and hyperammonemia excreted large amounts of argininosuccinic acid (ASA) and its anhydrides in urine (patient 2). The diagnosis of argininemia and argininosuccinic aciduria respectively was confirmed enzymatically by Dr. Bachmann in Bern. Both patients died soon after the diagnosis before the treatment was in effect.

We have developed sensitive radioactive methods for arginase (AG) and argininosuccinic lyase assays in order to study the characteristics of these enzymes further. A Column chromatographic procedure was designed for separation of three metabolites, arginine, ASA and urea using a mini Dowex column (0.6 x 1.0 cm). The AG activity was determined by measuring the synthesis of urea from $^{14}$C-arginine. The AG activity was deficient in erythrocytes and in leukocytes of the patient 1. The specific activity of AG in human tissues was very high (in erythrocytes, app. 3 mmol/h/g Hb; liver, app. 10 µmol/min/mg protein), somewhat higher than that determined by the conventional colorimetric method. The affinity for arginine of AG.(app. 10mM) was rather low in comparison with that of ASA lyase. Since ASA lyase is reversible, we have determined the activity by measuring the synthesis of ASA from fumaric acid and $^{14}$C-arginine (ASAS) and compared it with that by the conventional method of determination of the breakdown of ASA (AL). The normal values of ASAS in human tissues were app. 10-20 times higher than those of AL (liver, 300 vs. 15; kidney, 25 vs. 2). There was about 20% of the residual ASAS activity in the liver of patient 2, contrary to the reports of AL in which the activity was 0 among patients. However, the $K_m$ values for arginine of ASAS in the liver of the patient was much higher than normal (5.0 vs. 0.35 mM). In the kidney, however, a normal ASAS activity was obtained from patient 2 which is in agreement with the results of the AL assay.

In view of the severity of these aberrations and also the possible damages in utero it would be desirable to perform prenatal diagnosis.

LATE DIAGNOSIS OF AND THERAPEUTICAL APPROACH TO THE HYPERAMMONEMIA-HYPERORNITHINEMIA-HOMOCITRILLINURIA SYNDROME

*Otten, A., Bürger, U., Bachmann, C., Hillig, U., Wolf, H.*

Dep. of Pediatrics, Universities of Giessen and Bern, D-6300 Giessen, FRG

The hyperammonemia-hyperornithinemia-homocitrullinuria (HHH)-Syndrome is related to a disturbance of the urea cycle. The primary defect is not known. In view of the small numer of described patients, we would like to report the late diagnosis of HHH-Syndrome in two siblings and describe our therapeutical efforts.

At time of examination the 15 year-old boy appeared physically normal. His behavior was aggressive. His learning capability in school had deteriorated in the last two years (I.Q. 104). The 17 year old sister is tetraspastic and mentally retarded (I.Q. < 30). The regression of her development started at the age of 5-6 years. Both patients have a history of recurrent vomiting in early infancy. The boy refused to eat meat and milk products.

Analysis for detection of a metabolic disorder revealed slightly elevated blood ammonia (boy 50 µmol/l; girl 60 µmol/l) and high plasma ornithine levels (520 µmol/l; 312 µmol/l. An abnormal urinary excretion of homocitrulline was found (242 µmol; 260 µmol/g creatinine). Elevated blood ammonia concentrations and increased excretion of orotic acid (200 - 300 fold) confirmed the diagnosis of HHH-Syndrome.

Therapeutical efforts included restriction of protein and supplementation with arginine and/or citrulline (50 mg/kg body weight). The final diet contained 1,2 g/kg b.w. protein and citrulline. Metabolic parameters have normalised. To date, no significant clinical improvement has occured. Biochemical studies in search of the primary defect are underway.

# RELATIONSHIP BETWEEN DIETARY PHENYLALANINE TOLERANCE AND BIOCHEMICAL PARAMETERS OF THE ESTIMATION OF PHENYLALANINE HYDROXYLASE ACTIVITY

*Dhondt, J.-L., Farriaux, J.-P.*

Centre Régional de Dépistage des Maladies Métaboliques de l'Enfant.Institut Pasteur, Lille, France

For the last 10 years the heterogenity of hyperphenylalaninemic syndromes has became evident. Classic Phenylketonuria and Hyperphenylalaninemia are differentiated in regard to the intensity of the metabolic block and because of the decision on dietary treatment. Many parameters have been proposed to facilitate such a differential diagnosis. The aim of this work was to reconsider biochemical data obtained from 38 patients in order to establish what is the best parameter for the classification of the hyperphenylalaninemic patients. Parameters which have been selected are: neonatal blood phenylalanine concentration at the neonatal period, the course of blood phenylalanine under a standardized diet or following an oral phenylalanine load, and in vitro phenylalanine hydroxylase activity. All the patients of this study initially required a phenylalanine restricted diet on the basis of values of blood phenylalanine above 15 mg/dl on a normal proteic diet at the time of diagnosis. Thus, transient and mild hyperphenylalaninemias were exculded.
Patients have been retrospectively distributed into two groups : a group of 18 patients whose dietary tolerance (mg/d) remained low without significant variation with age and a group of 20 patients whose tolerance increased rapidly during the first year of treatment. Statistical comparison of the parameters from these two groups revealed that only the maximal blood phenylalanine concentration observed on a 180 mg/kg phenylalanine diet (at 6 months of age) was significantly different (Mann Whitney test). However, an important overlap between data from the 2 groups did not allow individual tolerance predictions. In vitro phenylalanine hydroxylase residual activity or data from oral phenylalanine load did not differentiate the two groups.

It remains clear that a wide heterogenity of phenylalanine hydroxylase deficiencies exist. High or increasing dietary tolerance is evidently related to an in vivo residual phenylalanine hydroxylase activity; however, such an anticipation is not always possible by simple biochemical investigation at the time of diagnosis and requires frequent evaluation during the first years of treatment.

# EVALUATION OF ORAL L-CYSTEINE FOR TREATMENT OF CYSTINE DEFICIENCY IN HOMOCYSTINURIA

*Byrd, D.J., Heinbokel, H., Schweitzer, S., Brodehl, J.*

Kinderklinik, Zentrum für Kinderheilkunde und Humangenetik, Medizinische Hochschule Hannover, Konstanty-Gutschow-Straße 8, 3000 Hannover 61, FRG

Homocystinuria (cystathionine synthase deficiency) is characterized by high plasma levels of methionine and homocystine and low levels of cystine (Cys). Supplements of Cys in the methionine free diet are recommended as treatment. In a 14 year old male patient with homocystinuria oral substitution with L-Cys (17 mg/kg/day) was therefore tried, but without success. Oral therapy with L-cysteine (1/2 Cys) and L-cysteine. HCI (1/2 Cys-HCI) was then considered to improve plasma Cys levels. Firstly, in a group of 10 healthy controls oral loading with 1/2 Cys and 1/2 Cys. HCI (49 mg/kg b.w.) as free amino acids and as components of a therapeutic methionine-free amino acid preparation increased plasma Cys from an average of 40 to 95 µmol/l after 90 min while Cys loading had no effect. The effect of oral free 1/2 Cys and 1/2 Cys. HCI was similar in the patient. Plasma Cys increased from 14 to 75 µmol/l in 105 min. The patient now receives 1/2 Cys.HCI in a dose of 8,5 mg/kg/day. His plasma Cys has increased over a period of 5 months from 22.8 $\pm$ 11. µmol/l to 50 $\pm$ 2.8 µmol/l.

In rats L-Cys and 1/2 Cys both increase plasma Cys after i.p. injection (0.8 µmol/kg). However the increase is greater by a factor of 6.5 when Cys is injected (66 vs.433 µmol/l at 15 min after injection). The parenterally administered 1/2 Cys is converted to taurine at a fast rate. The mechanism ba which enterally administered 1/2 Cys escapes rapid conversion to taurine and is able to argument plasma Cys is not yet understood. It is concluded that the rate of intestinal absorption of Cys is too slowto affect plasma Cys levels in the patient. The acute oral loading with 1/2 Cys was followed by an increase in the plasma concentration of the mixed disulfide of cysteine and homocysteine from 53 to 137 µmol/l after 30 min. The concentration remained elevated at 104.1 + 16.8 µmol/l during the following 90 min. Simultaneously the homocystine level fell from 65 to a minimum of 42 µmol/l at 120 min. This may indicate that some of the cysteine was incorporated into the mixed disulfide and caused a reduction in the plasma homocystine concentration.

## NUTRITIONAL CONTROL IN PKU CHILDREN ON RESTRICTED DIET: THE TRACE ELEMENTS

*Longhi, R., Riva, E., Rottoli, A., Paccanelli, S., Buttè, C., Valsasina, R., Giovannini, M.*

Clinica Pediatrica V Universita di Milano. Ospedale S. Paolo.
via Di Rudini 8. 20142 Milano. Italy

Serum copper and zinc levels were measured in 19 treated phenylketonuric (PKU) patients, as a part of the program of nutritional control undertaken by the V Pediatric Department of the University of Milan in order to point out the pathologies caused by liminal or selective malnutrition in patients on a restricted diet. These patients were in fact on a semisynthetic diet very low in phenylalanine. Serum copper and zinc levels were compared with those found in a group of 23 children in good health, on a normal diet. The minerals were determinated by atomic absorption spectrophotometry. The determinations were done in duplicate, reading against previously prepared standards. Statistical analyses were performed using Student's test for independent data whenever possible, and Mann and Whitney's U test. No differences were seen when the patients were devided by sex.
Plasma copper values were significantly lower in treated PKU patients than in the control population. At the dosage chosen, copper supplementation of PKU patients did not seem to be effective, since it did not cause an increase of the blood copper levels. Plasma zinc levels were also significantly lower in treated PKU patients than in normal subjects. This is even more evident in the patients in good metabolic control, presenting lower plasma phenylalanine values (and obviously on a stricter dietary regimen) and in those with good physical development.
Zinc supplementation influences the significance of the results because, while non supplemented PKU patients presented plasma zinc levels significantly lower than the controls, no differences could be noticed between the supplemented PKU and control groups.

## ZINC STATUS OF HISTIDINEMIC PATIENTS

*Matsuda, I., Kitano, A., Higashi, A., Nagata, N., Hase, Y.*

Department of Pediatrics, Kumamoto University Medical School,
Department of Pediatrics Ohsaka Children`s Medical Center

It was reported that oral administration of large amounts of L-histidine to man produced decreases in serum zinc concentration and increases in urinary zinc concentration (Henkin et al, Arch.Neurol 32:745, 1975). We measured zinc and histidine levels in serum, red blood cells, urine and hair samples in histidinemic patients. Carbonic anhydrase activity of red blood cells, which is one of the zinc-metalloenzyme was also measured. The results are shown in the table. In five out of 20 patients hair samples contained zinc levels lower than 80ug/g, but no one in controls. This observation proposed the possibility that histidinemia causes chronic zinc deficiency in some patients. (Humbidge: Pediat Clinc North Am 27:255, 1980).

Table Zinc and histidine levels in histidinemic patients

| | Control (N=15) | Patients(N=20) |
|---|---|---|
| Serum histidine (μmol/dl) | 9.6 ± 4.5 | *52.9 ± 30.9 |
| Serum Zinc (μg/ml) | 0.99± 0.24 | 0.93± 0.18 |
| Red blood cell histidine (μmole/gHb) | 1.3 ± 0.4 | * 2.6 ± 0.5 |
| Red blood cell zinc (μg/gHb) | 29.1 ± 6.9 | 31.7 ± 11.7 |
| Red blood cell cargonic anhydrase (U/gHb) | 10.1 ± 1.4 | 10.2 ± 1.4 |
| Urine histidine (μmol/mgCr) | 0.85± 0.3 | * 4.7 ± 1.5 |
| Urine zinc (mg/gCr) | 1.1 ± 0.3 | ** 2.2 ± 1.1 |
| Hair zinc (μg/g) | 152.9 ±81.8 | 129 ± 15.5 |
| below 80ug/g | 0/10 | 5/20 |

* p<0.01 **p<0.05

ANDERSONS'S DISEASE : AN INBORN ERROR OF INTESTINAL LIPID TRANSPORT

*Infante, R., Beucler, I., Bouma, M.E., Schmitz*, J., Amit, N.*

INSERM U 9, Hôpital Saint-Antoine and Gastroenterology Clinic, Hôpital des Enfants Maldes*, Paris - France

Since the former description in 1961 by ANDERSON et al. of an unusual case of infantile steatorrhoea associated with absence of postprandial chylomicronemia and low levels of apo-B containing plasma lipoproteins several similar cases have been reported in the literature. The molecular defect involved in the disease is still unknown.
Three new cases have been thoroughly investigated. Specifically, plasma lipoprotein composition and structure in a basal state and after feeding a fat-enriched diet and production of apo-lipoprotein B by the intestine have been studied.
The children presented with typical coeliac-like syndrome, steatorrhoea, and failure to thrive. Plasma lipoproteins were isolated by ultracentrifugation and their lipid and apoprotein composition was determined by conventional methods. Jejunal mucosa samples obtained by tube biopsy were studied by general and fat-staining techniques ; mucosa fragments were dissociated by WEISER` s technique in order to obtain isolated villous cells : neutral fat (Oil Red) and apoprotein-B (immunoperoxidase) were stained by specific methods. After overnight fast, plasma cholesterol was 30-50 % of normal values and triglyceride was in the lower normal range. Apo-AI 20-50 % and apo B 30-50 % of normal levels. Any of these abnormally low values were significantly raised 3 h after a fat-rich meal ; lipoprotein lipid and apoprotein patterns were not modified by fat ingestion substantiating a lack of production of chylomicron or other intestinal lipoproteins. The intestinal form of apoprotein B (apo-B-48) was absent from fasting and postprandial plasma. Interestingly, however villous intestinal cells of these children contained huge amounts of apo-B reacting with peroxidase-labeled antibodies. Intestinal cells had a normal structure and shape, and the brush border height was not reduced. All the cells were heavily loaded with Oil- Red-stained neutral fat droplets mainly located above the nucleus, a picture ressembling those observed in mucosa biopsies from abetalipoproteinemia patients, a genetically determined deletion of apoprotein-B synthesis. These results bring new insigth on the molecular mechanisms of Anderson`s disease;

namely, they demonstrate that it is not due to defective production of intestinal apoprotein-B (necessary to chylomicron formation). Whether a defective lipid-apoprotein packaging or an impaired secretion of normal chylomicron is the primary defect responsible for fat malabsorption in Anderson's disease, remains to be elucidated.

## DIFFERENCES IN INDIVIDUAL RESPONSE OF SERUM CHOLESTEROL TO DIETARY CHOLESTEROL IN RATS, RABBITS AND MAN

*Beynen*[1,2], *A.C.*, *Katan*[1], *M.B.*, *van Zutphen*[2], *L.F.M.*

1)Dept. of Human Nutrition, Agricultural Univ., 6703 BC Wageningen
[2]Dept. of Laboratory Animal Science, Univ. of Utrecht, 3508 TD Utrecht
(The Netherlands)

Differences in the response of serum cholesterol to dietary cholesterol in rabbits and rats have a genetic basis. In inbred rabbits a 5-fold greater response was found in two hyper-responsive strains than in two hypo-response strains. Similar differences in serum cholesterol response between inbred strains of rats were also observed.
The inheritance of the response was studied in male rats from crosses between hyper- and hypo-responding strains. Comparison of the variances of the response of genetically uniform groups (parental strains and $F_1$ hybrid) and segregating groups (backcrosses and $F_2$ hybrid) revealed that more than 80 percent of the observed variation was due to additive genetic factors, and that two major genes are involved in the control of the serum cholesterol response.
We have carried out three controlled dietary trials with the same subjects to see whether humans exist with a consistently high or low serum cholesterol response to an increase in cholesterol intake from about 120 to 650 mg/day. Fifteen putative hypo- and 17 hyper-responders with mean serum cholesterol increases of -0.01 and 0.96 mmol/l were selected in the first experiment and participated in the second and third trial. Although the response in each individual was only partly reproducible from one study to another, the hyper-responders consistently showed a significantly higher serum cholesterol response in the second and third trial than did the selected hypo-responders. We conclude that human hyper- and hypo-responders do exist, and it is now important to investigate whether the cholesterolemic response in man is genetically determined as has been shown in rabbits and rats. Supported by grant no.

31.013 of the Netherlands Heart Foundation and an established investigatorship to M.B.K.

SYSTEMIC CARNITINE DEFICIENCY (SDC) IN TWO ADULT SISTERS: FULL RECOVERY WITH L-CARNITINE SUPPLEMENTATION.

*Di Donato, S., Pelucchetti, D., Rimoldi, M.*

Istituto Neurologico "C. Besta", Via Celoria 11, 20133 Milan, Italy

SDC is characterized clinically by recurrent episodes of metabolic acidosis and encephalopathy associated with progressive muscular weakness (Karpati et al.,1975 ). It is inherited as an autosomal recessive trait (Di Donato et al., 1982) and usually develops in infancy or childhood. Two sisters had, at age 19 and 21 respectively, episodes of nausea and vomiting. Subsequently, they developed progressive muscular weakness and wasting. The older girl had respiratory insufficiency. Muscle and liver biopsies showed in both accumulation of lipid droplets: the mitochondria had normal appearance. Total carnitine content was 4.4 and 4.7 nanomoles/mg non collagen protein (ncp) in the patients` muscles 2.8 and 2.2 nanomoles/mg ncp in the patients` livers and 29.1 and 32.1 nanomoles/ml respectively in the patients` plasma. Carnitine values in 36 non-weak controls were 21.1 $\pm$ 1.1 (SD) nanomoles/mg ncp in muscle, 11.5 $\pm$ 1.2 SD nanomoles/mg ncp in liver and 53.4 $\pm$ 2.0 nanomoles/ml in plasma. Biochemical studies of cultured fibroblasts, skeletal muscle mitochondria and biological fluids from the two sisters showed no evidence of other genetic diseases that might deplete tissue carnitine stores. Carnitine supplementation (4 g L-carnitine per os, dayly) dramaticly improved their clinical conditions. They rapidly gained weight and strength and lipid droplets disappeared from their muscles. Total plasma carnitine rose, after 4 months of supplementation, to 59.2 and 56.7 nanomoles/ml; muscle carnitine rose to 10.3 and 11.4 nanomoles/mg ncp respectively. This form of systemic carnitine deficiency, that might be due to defective carnitine biosynthesis, is an example of treatable inherited metabolic disease.

- Karpati G., Carpenter S., Engel AG et al.:Neurology 25: 16-24, 1975.
- Di Donato S., Rimoldi M., Cornelio F et al.: Ann.Neurol. 11:190-92, 1982.

CLINICAL VARIABILITY OF MATURITY-ONSET TYPE DIABETES OF YOUNG PEOPLE (MODY)

*Füessl, H.S., Goebel, F.-D.*

Medizinische Poliklinik der Universität, Pettenkoferstraße 8 a, 8000 München 2. FRG.

According to te criteria of Tattersall (1974) MODY has been regarded as a disorder of carbohydrate metabolism with dominant inheritance and benign course compared to juvenile-onset diabetes (JOD). Only a few case reports of late complications in MODY-diabetics have been published.
With a 24 year old female as proposita having a history of intermittent glucosuria since her 9th year and several follow-up abnormal glucose tolerance tests a complete family study was conducted. 30 family members in 5 generations were diabetics. The course of the disease was heterogeneous. 20 diabetics did not show any late complications even with diabetes up to 40 years duration. 6 patients had severe complications such as diabetic coma and late sequelae such as proliferative retinopathy and nephropathy with renal failure. Tissue typing did not reveal linkage between HLA and MODY.
Thus, MODY seems to be a disease of great clinical variability in spite of dominant inheritance. Late complications in MODY are more infrequent than in JOD but they can occur. This suggests the need of lifelong metabolic control in MODY.

DIAGNOSIS OF VARIOUS TYPES OF GLYCOGEN STORAGE DISEASES WITH BLOOD SAMPLES. INCREASED AMYLO-1,6 - $\alpha$ - GLUCOSIDASE ACTIVITY IN ERTHROCYTES IN GLYCOGENOSIS VIa

*Shin, Y.S., Ullrich*, K., Kopp, H., Rieth, M., v.Rücker, A., Endres, W.*

Children's Hospital, Univ. of Munich, München, FRG
*Children's Hospital, Univ. of Münster, Münster, FRG

It is a common practice to perform biopsy for the diagnosis of most types of glycogen storage diseases. The former procedure is rather unpleasant and the shipment of the analysing materials is also time-consuming and troublesome. Therefore we have tried to develop a sensitive methodology in order to do diagnosis with materials as little as possible as well as with easily accessible samples such as heparinized blood. Diagnosis of various glycogenoses, type II (lysosomal α-glucosidase deficiency), type III (debranching enzyme def.) and type VIa (phosphorylase b kinase def.) can be perfomed by the respective enzyme assays and measurement of glycogen in erythrocytes or in leukocytes. In the case of type II it is possible by the determination of the specific isoenzyme with the aid of antibodies for liver acid α-glucosidase (homozygotes, 0-0.2 nmol/min/mg protein; normal, 0.7-2.5). With a simplified procedure for glycogen purification one can easily assay various enzymes by monitoring the incorporation of the respective substrates into glycogen; $^{14}$C-glucose for type III, $^{14}$C-glucose-1-phosphate for the phosphorylase assay and UDP-$^{14}$C-glucose for glycogen synthase and branching enzyme assays. An extreme increase in glycogen concentrations in erythrocytes was found in glycogenosis type III and type VIa (68-630 mg/100 ml) in comparison with normal erythrocytes (up to 9 mg). Interestingly enough the amylo-1,6-α-glycosidase activity significantly increased in erythrocytes of patients with phosphorylase b kinase deficiency (30-70 nmol glucose incorporated/min/g Hb; normal, 10-21). This may be due to a compensatory action of gluconeogenesis and in any case would certainly help to confirm the diagnosis of type VIa. Further studies concerning the diagnosis of other glycogen storage diseases, i.e., type IV (branching enzyme def.), type VIb (liver phosphorylase def.) and type VII (phosphofructokinase def.) are in progress.

## TREATMENT OF DEFECTS IN BIOPTERIN METABOLISM

*Berlow, S., Hoganson*, G., Kaufman[+], S., Muenzer,[+] J.*

*University of Wisconsin, Madison, Wisconsin
[+]National Institutes of Health, Bethesda, Maryland, USA

The recognition that biopterin synthesis defects (BSD) and dihydropteridine reductase (DHPR) deficiency can cause neonatal hyperphenylalaninemia, has given impetus to the early identification of these conditions, with the expectation that treatment might prevent serious CNS manifestations. The studies which we will report were perfomed in two subjects with different BSD. In an asymptomatic newborn, we have tried to define the nature of the defect in order to be certain that therapy was indeed required. We have also treated a 13 year old boy, a "leaky" mutant for BSD., with different therapies in an effort to determine optimal therapy.

Our studies employed plasma phenylalanine (phe) and tyrosine determinations. Biopterin and neopterin were measured in urine, plasma and CSF. Catecholamines (CA) and neutrotransmitter (NT) metabolites were measured in CSF. An activity meter was employed to monitor movement and psychological evaluations were used to assess developmental progress.

The newborn hyperphenylalaninemic infant had elevated neopterin and low biopterin in urine and plasma. Oral tetrahydrobiopterin ($BH_4$) lowered plasma phe levels to normal. CSF neopterin, biopterin and NT metabolites were normal throughout the study. Since the age of 2 months, the infant has received no treatment; at age 18 months her growth and development were normal.

Studies which have been reported elsewhere, in the boy who is a "leaky" BSD mutant, will be briefly reviewed as a background for data now presented. From age 7-11 years, while on DOPA and 5-hydroxytryptophan, he made developmental progress at a delayed rate. During his 11th year, he was given, in separate trials, oral $BH_4$ or 6-methyltetrahydropterin ($6MPH_4$) at 20 mg/kg/day. With both neurological pterins, there was marked improvement in symptoms, the improvement with $6MPH_4$ being documented with an activity meter. The use of $6MPH_4$ was stopped when serum levels of hepatic enzymes increased. Re-institution of DOPA and 5HT therapy was associated, after 3 months, with loss of drug effectiveness.

We conclude that the heterogenity of defects in biopterin metabolism requires not only precision in neonatal pterin screening but also confirmation of CNS involvement, demonstrated by CSF analyses of CA and/or NT metabolites-before institution of therapy. $BH_4$response, measured by phe levels, is inadequate evidence alone, on which to start treatment.

We also conclude that more studies, especially long-term clinical trials, are needed to define which treatment (s) is best for these different metabolic defects. It is hoped that the natural cofactor will prove to be more effective therapy. Although our preliminary results with pterin therapy for treatment of BSD are encouraging, further studies are required to determine whether the favorable response seen in this patient is persistent and general.

# **Short Communications,** Room C

FRIDAY, MARCH 9, 1984

LATE COMERS' SESSION II
Chairman: E. Siess (München/FRG)

| | |
|---|---|
| 9.00 | J. Zlotogora, G. Bach (Jerusalem)<br>Prenatal Diagnosis of Hunter Syndrome in Materalä Serum |
| 9.15 | I. Krieger, L.L. Bieber (Detroit)<br>Carnitine Metabolism in a Case of Dicarboxylic Aciduria (DC Auria) Due to Deficient Acetyl-CoA Disposal |
| 9.30 | G. Jacobasch, H.-G. Holzhütter (Berlin)<br>Mathematical Modelling of Glycolysis Affected by Pyruvate Kinase Deficiency |
| 9.45 | B. Molzer, H. Bernheimer, A. Roscher (Wien, Graz)<br>Accumulation of Very Long Chain Fatty Acids (VLFA) in Adrenoleucodystrophy (ALD) Variants |
| 10.00 | J. Lößner, H.-J. Kühn, J. Zotter, R. Siegemund, H. Bachmann, W. Storch, D. Biesold (Leipzig)<br>Therapeutic Approaches in Wilson's Disease |
| 10.15 | G. Spiteller (Bayreuth)<br>Individual Different Metabolism of Piperine |
| 10.30 | Coffee Break |
| 11.00 | Böhles, H.J., Lehnert, W. (Erlangen, Freiburg)<br>The Effect of L-carnitine on Propionic Acid Excretion in Acute Stage of Propionic Acidemia |
| 11.15 | Schlierf, G., Wirth, A. (Heidelberg/FRG)<br>Glycerokinase deficiency: Hyperglycerolemia, Glyceroluria and Pseudohypertriglyceridemia |

PRENATAL DIAGNOSIS OF HUNTER SYNDROME IN MATERNAL SERUM

*Zlotogaora, J., Bach, G.*

Department of Human Genetics ,Hadassah University Hospital, Jerusalem, Israel

Hunter syndrome, an x-linked recessive disorder, is caused by the deficiency of the lysosomal hydrolase iduronate sulfate (ISS). A sensitive assay technique of this enzyme in serum enabled us to detect over 90 % of obligatory heterozygotes for this disorder. Enzyme values per individual were relatively constant in repeated determinations and no significant changes were observed in relation to sex or age. In control women, during pregnancy a consistant increase of ISS activity in serum was noted, approaching a four fold increase before delivery. In four pregnant Hunter carriers, whose initial ISS values were in the heterozygote range, a similar increase of enzyme activity was noted when the fetus was not affected by Hunter disease. This increase in ISS activity was noted in maternal serum as early as the 12th week of the pregnancy. On the other hand, in a second pregnancy of one of these carriers, a Hunter affected fetus was diagnosed and then the enzyme activity remained unaltered until the termination of the pregnancy at the 21st week of the pregnancy. In the precedent pregnancy with the normal fetus ISS increased in the serum of this women already at the 17th week. These results indicate a correlation between the state of the fetus with regard to Hunter syndrome and ISS activity in maternal serum so that this test might be used for prenatal diagnosis of this disorder.
These findings are in accordance to the relatively high concentrations of this enzyme in the amniotic fluid and the known transfer of proteins from the amniotic fluid to the maternal serum.

CARNITINE METABOLISM IN A CASE OF DICARBOXYLIC ACIDURIA (DC-Auria) DUE TO DEFICIENT ACETYL-CoA DISPOSAL

*Krieger, I., Bieber, L.L.*

Wayne State Univ. Detroit, Mich. and Michigan State Univ. E. Lansing. Mich., USA

A 10 month old infant had 3 Reye Syndrome-like attacks with elevated $NH_4$ (158 µg/dl) and SGOT (312 µU/ml). He excreted large amounts of ß-hydroxybutyrate and acetoacetate and the following DCA's: adipate, suberate, sebacate, ethylmalonate and moderate glutarate. Production of $CO_2$ from ($1-^{14}C$) and ($U-^{14}C$) palmitate and ($1-^{14}C$) butyrate by cultured fibroblasts was 83 %, 5 % and 50 % of normal, respectively.Acyl-CoA dehydrogenase activity in fibroblasts was normal. Analysis of individual short-chain acylcarnitines (SCAC) in urine revealed disproportionately high excretion of acetylcarnitine (152 µmol/gr creat.). The DCAuria was eliminated by continuous i.v. glucose infusion and exaggerated by fasting and a ketogenic diet containing MCT-oil. Moderate DCA excretion persisted after recovery on a low protein-low fat diet, but disappeared completely on riboflavin therapy (100 mg/day). Inspite of the apparent treatment response, the patient developed within 2 month generalized hypotonia. Plasma carnitine had dropped from 22.2 µmol/l during the attack to 14.4 µmol/l (normal 41.5). Carnitine metabolism was therefore studied. Total urinary carnitine was normal during the attack, but the ratio of SCAC to free carnitines was increased. This ratio is believed to mirror the ratio of acyl-CoA/CoA-SH. Consequently, CoA-SH appeared to be trapped as acyl-CoA because of carnitine deficiency. Treatment with oral carnitine did indeed cause massive excretion of SCAC (994 µmol/gr creat.), which continued in that range carnitine, 620 µmol/gr creat., which is similar to values seen in adults after 60 hrs. starvation! These ovservation show that the risk of carnitine deficiency is high in disorders of ß-oxidation or acetyl-CoA disposal because of chronis urinary SCAC loss which is not reflected in deficient patients by absolute urine values. The response to carnitine treatment indicates that carnitine modulates the intramitochondrial acyl-CoA/CoA-SH ratio and - by freeing CoA-SH - may prevent Reye Syndrome-like attacks.

## MATHEMATICAL MODELLING OF GLYCOLYSIS AFFECTED BY PYRUVATE KINASE DEFICIENCY

*Jacobasch*, G., *Holzhütter*, H.-G.

Inst. of Physiol. & Biol. Chem., Humboldt Univ., DDR 1040 Berlin, Hessische Str. 3/4

The mathematical model of glycolysis takes into account the main regulatory properties of the nonequilibrium enzymes and the magnesium-complex formation by the adenine nucleotides and 2,3-$P_2$G. PK deficiency leads to a remarkable decrease of the glycolytic flux and the ATP concentration of about 50 % of a normal control. The control strength of the deficient PK increases and can become fluxlimiting.

Heterozygotes exhibit no significant changes of the metabolite concentrations and the flux rates compared with normal values which is in accordance with the lack of clinical symptoms.
For three probands with known changes of the kinetic properties of their PK mutants the calculated metabolite concentrations and the control characteristics permit to estimate the degree of disorder of the glycolytic pathway. The resulting classification corresponds well with other independent and clinical findings. The calculation demonstrates that there are no simple correlations between the decreased enzyme activity and the reduced flux rate through the affected pathway.

## ACCUMULATION OF VERY LONG CHAIN FATTY ACIDS (VLFA) IN ADRENOLEUKODYSTROPHY (ALD) VARIANTS

*Molzer*[1], B., *Bernheimer*[1], H., *Roscher*[2], A.

[1]Neurological Insitute, Univ. Vienna, Schwarzspanierstr. 17, A-1090 Vienna, and
[2]Department of Pediatrics, Univ. Graz, Austria

ALD is an X-linked recessively inherited disease with central nervous system (CNS) demyelonation and adrenocortical atrophy. 4 ALD variants may be differentiated: "classical" ALD (boys), adrenomyeloneuropathy (AMN; male juveniles and adults), "atypical" ALD (females of different age, probably heterozygotes) and neonatal (connatal) ALD (possibly inherited as autosomal recessive trait). Biochemically, increase of VLFA ($>$ 24C), mainly of C26:0, is found in certain lipids of CNS white matter (WM), peripheral tissues, and blood, probably due to an enzyme deficiency in the peroxisomal β-oxidation of fatty acids. Neurochemical data on ALD variants, however, were incomplete.
We analyzed VLFA of CNS WM cholesterol esters in classical ALD (n=7), AMN (n=2), atypical (n=4) and connatal (n=1) ALD. Increased percentages of VLFA (16.4–71.7%) were found in the ALD material as compared with controls (n=18; 0.4–14.3%). The major accumulation VLFA was C26:0 (ALD: 3.6–26.0%; controls: 0–1.4%). Thus, accumulation of VLFA, particularly of C26:0 in WM cholesterol esters is a common marker for all ALD variants. Investigations of WM gangliosides revealed increase of C24:0 in classical (n=4), atypical (n=4), and connatal (n=1) ALD, but not in AMN (n=2). With regard to the clinical chemical diagnosis of ALD estimation of C26:0 concentrations in leukocytes (preferably granulocytes?), in addition to fibroblasts or serum, may be important.

Recently, an accumulation of C26:0 in certain CNS and peripheral lipids was found also in Zellweger's cerebro-hepato-renal syndrome (ZS; Brown et al., Johns Hopkins Med. J. 151: 344, 1982), a disease due to deficiency of peroxisomes. We confirmed C26:0 accumulation in ZS fibroblasts (n=3). Moreover, we observed an increase of VLFA with a tetention time near to C26:1, a finding not detectable in fibroblasts from classical (n=3) or neonatal (n=1) ALD. Therefore, biochemical discrimination between ZS and ALD might be possible also by VLFA analysis in fibroblasts.

(Supported by Austrian Science Research Fund, Projekt Nr. S-25/04).

## THERAPEUTIC APPROACHES IN WILSON'S DISEASE

*Lössner, J., Kühn, H.-J., Zotter, J., Siegemund*[+]*, R., Bachmann, H., Storch, W., Biesold, D.*

Neurologic Clinic and Dept. of Neurochemistry, Paul Flechsig Institute of Brain Research[+], Karl Marx University, Leipzig, GDR.

In Wilson's disease (hepatocerebral degeneration) the disturbed copper balance leading to an accumulation of this metal preferentially in liver, brain and kidney can be normalized by lifelong treatment with chelatin agents such as D-penicillamine removing the surplus of copper by excretion through the kidney. Improvements in the detection of this rare disease have been achieved in the GDR since 1970 by centralizing at our departments in Leipzig the diagnostic investigations including the search for so-called asymptomatic cases within affected families, the control of the effects of the treatment and the rehabilitation. Some clinics took over the after-care of the confirmed cases.
In the GDR within the last 15 years 174 cases with Wilson's disease including asymptomatic cases have been detected. In all asymptomatic cases and in most patients with clinical symptoms the long-term treatment with D-penicillamine was of great benefit preventint the occurrence of clinical symptoms in the first group and normalizing the disturbing effect of copper accumulation in both groups. However, in 20 % of the 51 patients being in long-term care of our clinic the development of harmful side-effects of D-penicillamine of toxic or immunopathological origin became obviously. From these side-effects the nephrotic syndrome and the immunocomplexnephritis were of special interest.
According to recommendations in the literature in these patients D-penicillamine can be substituted by triethylene tetramine dihydrochloride (triene) or zinc

sulphate. In 4 patients we applied triene in a dosage of 1200 mg/day over a period of one year, 8 patients received zinc sulphate in a dosage of 600 mg/day over a period of three years. No clinical or laboratory side-effects were observed with both drugs, and no reoccurrence of clinical symptoms became obviously. From the copper excretion through the kidney triene seems to be a valuable substitute of D-penicillamine, whereas zins sulphate does not normalize the copper balance adequately.

## INDIVIDUAL DIFFERENT METABOLISM OF PIPERINE

*Hölzel, C., Spiteller, G.,*

Univ. Bayreuth, Postf. 3008, Organische Chemie I, 8580 Bayreuth

In the course of an investigation of steroids in urine by gas-chromatography-mass spectrometry one disturbing peak in the gas-chromatograms revealed the presence of a previously unknown compound.
This compound could be enriched in respect to the steroids by short time encymatic hydrolysis (10 min). High resolution mass spectrometry allowed the structural assignment to this compound, confirmed later by synthesis, to be 1. A second interfering peak in the steroid profiles was shown to have structure 2. 1 show some relationship to piperine 3, the active principle of pepper. If nutrition free of pepper was eaten 1 and 2 disappeared in the gas-chromatograms and appeared again after intake of 3. Therefore 1 and 2 are metabolites of 3. 1 and 2 were not found in the profiles of some people. If these people were feeded with large doses of pepper a third and forth metabolite was found, 5 and 6, present in pepper-non-metabolizers only in trace amounts.
Out of 20 persons 2 were not able to metabolize pepper to 1 and 2, but only to 4 and 5. From one of the non-metabolizers urine samples were available also from a daughter and a son. The daughter was shown to be a non-metabolizer, the son turned out to be able to produce 1 and 2 besides 4 and 5.

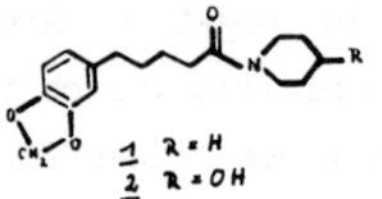

1 R = H
2 R = OH

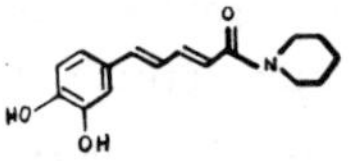

3

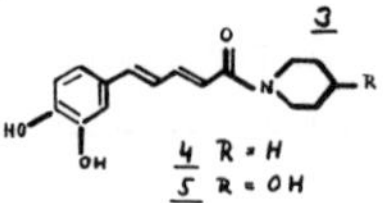

4 R = H
5 R = OH

THE EFFECT OF L-CARNITINE ON PROPIONIC ACID EXCRETION IN ACUTE STAGE OF PROPIONIC ACIDEMIA

*Böhles*[1], H.J., *Lehnert*[2], W.

[1]Universitätskinderklinik Erlangen; [2]Universitätskinderklinik Freiburg

A six week old female infant was presented in a severe metabolic crisis from propionic acidemia. The condition was aggravated by pneumonia and heart insufficiency. Additionally to the general supportive measures and caloric intake exclusively from glucose, intravenous L-carnitine treatment (2 g L-carnitine / 24 hours) was started in order to enhance propionic acid excretion as a carnitine conjugate. Despite of the therapeutic efforts the patient died about 48 hours after admission in sudden respiratory arrest and bradycardia. Serum propionic acid concentration was increased to 0.3 µmol/ml. Propionylcarnitine excretion was measured and about 55 % of the over all excretion during the 48 hour treatment period were attributed to be an effect of carnitine administration. Obviously carnitine was not able to prevent metabolic deterioration, but it may provide some additional "buffer capacity" during long term dietary treatment.

GLYCEROKINASE DEFICIENCY: HYPERGLYCEROLEMIA, GLYCEROLURIA AND PSEUDOHYPERTRIGLYCERIDEMIA

*Wirth*, A., *Schlierf*, G.

Klinisches Institut für Herzinfakrtforschung an der Medizinischen Universitätsklinik Heidelberg, Heidelberg/FRG

Three men with glycerokinase deficiency were investigated under several conditions. Glycerol concentrations in serum were between 2.8 and 4.0 mMol/l glyceroluria amounted between 15 and 48 g/d. Glycerokinase deficiency was ascertained by converion of glycerol to glycerophosphate and the oxidation of $C^{14}$-glycerol to $CO_2$. Compared to controls the activity amounted from 6 to 18%. Moreover, an oral glycerol load indicated an impaired disappearance of glycerol from the circulation. All subjects were apparantly healthy as ascertained by a clinical laboratory check up.

Since gycerol is an important precurosr of glucose the subjects were studied under conditions of enhanced gluconeogenesis. Fasting up to 36h and bicycle exercise

up to 3h (even during fasting) did not induce hypoglycemia.
It is concluded that glycerokinase deficiency is going along with hyperglycerolemia and glyceroluria. Despite a marked reduction of gycerokinase activity gluconeogenesis is guaranteed even under conditions of enhanced glucose need. On the other hand the marked elevation of serum glycerol levels may lead to falsely high measured triglyceride concentrations.

Authors